IN PRAISE OF NO CHEATIN', JUST EATIN'

"*No Cheatin', Just Eatin'* shines a light on the struggles of yo-yo dieting and weight shame that too many of us share. Author Mary Jo Fay takes you on her journey from fit high school track team athlete, to getting way too close to 200 pounds, and finally doing something about it. Through heart-break, pain, tragedy and loss, to the carrot-dangling prize of being in shape for her daughter's wedding, we walk with her. We've been there. This book shows us a different way, a doable way to slim down and find the body we know is in there somewhere."

—Mary Catherine Carwile, speaker and award-winning author of "Heartstrings at 35,000 Feet"

"Once again, Mary Jo Fay knocks it out of the park with her new book about weight loss. Taking a new direction on the topic, she has cleverly mixed her own life of dieting ups and downs with new insights on how she eventually lost 40 pounds while eating anything she wanted. If you think you're the only one who has ever struggled with a diet and lost, you owe it to yourself to read this book. Highly recommended!"

—Judith Briles, the Book Shepherd

"*No Cheatin', Just Eatin'* is one of those rare books that most women will find themselves in, one way or another. Mary Jo Fay's journey shows us that all those weight loss goals many of us believe to be impossible due to our age, or a variety of other excuses, are just that – excuses."

—Joyce Leake, founder of Odd Duck Society

"Mary Jo tells the truth in a way that everyone can relate to; a down-to earth, honestly raw approach while sharing completely relatable stories you'll giggle about! We've all played the mind games she's played; she's just vulnerable and humble enough to expose her underbelly, a belly we all tend to hide in more ways than one! If you don't see your own weight or food struggle in hers, you're not human! Giddy up! This one's a doozy!"

—Laura Menze, Chief Love Officer, Ready-Match.com

"In my early 30s, I went through the big weight loss process. Although I have mostly maintained my weight over the last 20 years, this book has been a good reminder to me to be more mindful of my calories and what I'm putting in my mouth and why."

—Becky Drager, artist, DragerStudios.com

"As a former body builder constantly counting every morsel that went in my mouth, I can relate to this book in so many ways. Battling the shame of cheating, especially when the next competition was right around the corner, left me with so much guilt and anguish. What was almost harder was trying to let go of all those expectations once I was no longer competing. This book allowed me to realize that a lot of other people are affected by the obsession of wanting to look good and wanting a fast fix to obtain that. And just how much alike all of us are in our oftentimes frustrating journeys."

—Marjorie Collins, body builder

"The biggest lesson I learned from *No Cheatin', Just Eatin'* is that I can't outrun the fork! It's got 2 more legs than me! 'Nuf said!"

—Dianna Sumanas, Rocky Mountain Singles

"So you want to lose weight? Read this book! Forget about how you should eat this and not that, and so much other blah, blah, blah! Learn to approach food without guilt, take responsibility for your decisions, and make them your own. I've lost almost 10 lbs. in the last 3 months after reading it, and I do not feel guilty when I have another glass of wine or piece of chocolate. I get back on track and move forward. Thank you, Mary Jo Fay, for giving me the tools to make this my new life style."

—Nancy Stern, paralegal

"Mary Jo Fay teaches us that 'tryin's lyin' – especially when it comes to diets and weight loss. I look back at how many times I said I was going to "try" some new diet or other, never realizing that I was never fully vested in the diet to begin with. No wonder all those diets never worked!"

—Rene Ryman, PhD, Professor of International business

OTHER WORKS BY MARY JO FAY

GET OUT OF YOUR BOXX!

THE SEVEN SECRETS OF LOVE

PLEASE DEAR, NOT TONIGHT

BLATANT DECEPTION

WHEN YOUR PERFECT PARTNER GOES PERFECTLY WRONG

No Cheatin', Just Eatin'

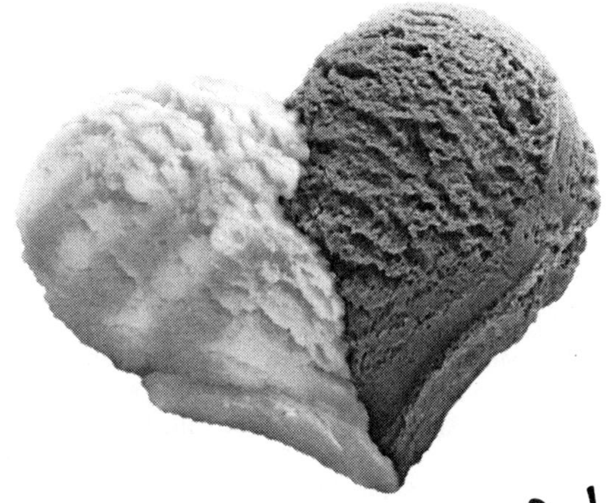

My ~~crazy~~ successful love/hate relationship with food

Mary Jo Fay

Out of the Boxx, Inc.
Topeka, Kansas

NO CHEATIN', JUST EATIN'
by Mary Jo Fay

Published by

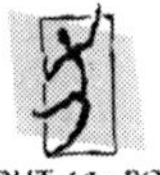

Books may be purchased in quantity by contacting the publisher directly.
OutOfTheBoxx.com
303-841-7691
OutOfTheBoxxInc@aol.com

Editing: Barb Munson, Munson Communications Editorial Services
Cover and Interior Design: Nick Zelinger, NZ Graphics
Author Photo: Margie LeBow

ISBN: 978-0-9981764-0-6 (paper)
ISBN: 978-0-9981764-1-3 (eBook)
Library of Congress Control Number: 2016917426

Disclaimer

This is my true story. Nothing I include in here is a recognized diet by any entity or company. In fact, it is a way of eating that likely no nutritionist or physician would approve of. I am not suggesting that you or anyone you love (or hate) eat this way. This is simply what worked, and continues to work, for me. As everyone is different, you might find that something totally different works better for you. This is not to be taken as medical advice. However, if you're already eating an unhealthy diet, filled with sugar, candy, chocolate, pizza, or whatever your food of choice is that has gotten you where you are now, it is my hope that at least it might help you make some smarter choices. See your doctor before beginning any new weight loss program.

Memoir. Self-help. Diet and Weight Loss.
First Edition
Printed in the United States

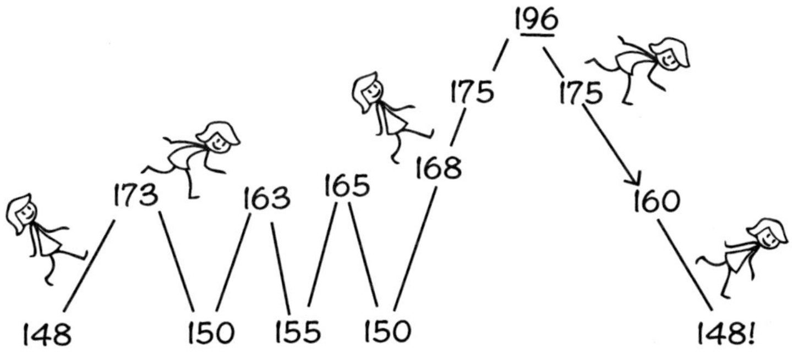

This book is dedicated to the pounds left behind
I just didn't want to carry anymore.

mary Jo Fay

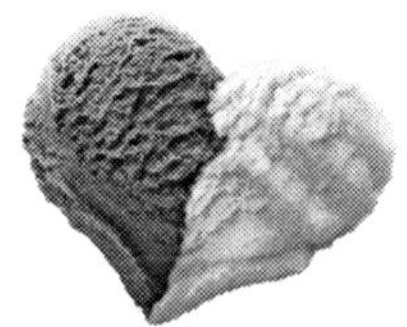

CHAPTER 1

Closet Sugar Junkie

Are you the kind of person who has battled your weight at least once in your life, if not all of your life? Do you feel surrounded by thin people everywhere? You know the ones I'm talking about; the ones with the great figures who you always see eating anything they want and never gaining weight.

You hate those people, right? It seems like you just look at food and you gain weight, while they never gain an ounce yet still bring that large Starbucks Mocha Latte and a couple of donuts to the office every day and, nope, never gain an inch around the middle, or anywhere else, for that matter.

Well, I'm here to share with you how not all those thin people are thin by nature. Many (and I was one of them) either struggle every day to keep their weight down or have actually lost weight and now they're thin, but it was a struggle for them as well. Yep, they did it. They know full-well what it's like to be overweight – but you may not be aware of their "before" stories. You may just assume that they magically keep the weight off because they're lucky or blessed or simply have a higher metabolism or better genetic code than you.

People treat me like that all the time, as though I've always been skinny. They don't realize that, while much of my life I was of average weight (I don't think I was ever skinny), I also tipped the scales at nearly 200 pounds several years back. Yep, 200 pounds. Now, while 200 pounds may not be obese, it was a good 40 pounds more than I needed to carry around. And I wonder just how many more pounds I might have ended up with, had I not made some changes.

Those extra 40 pounds meant that I didn't fit into my clothes, necessitating spending more and more money on increasingly roomier ones. Those extra 40 pounds also made it harder to walk fast without huffing and puffing. They made me feel like I looked pregnant, and to some I did.

I mean, trust me – you don't have to be 100 pounds overweight to wish you could shed some pounds. Many folks just need to lose those 10, 20, or 50 pounds to make a big difference in their health. In fact, something like two in three adults in the US are overweight or obese today. That extra 40 pounds put me in the Overweight category on my doctor's scales. Never thought I'd see *that* day!

But, granted, whether you want to lose 10 or 100 pounds, it's simply not easy. (If it were, everyone would be skinny, right?)

Well, I did my share of trying this diet and that diet, especially all the so-called fad diets that came and went. Some worked for a while – some never really worked at all. With most I didn't last more than a week or so. Weight Watchers was OK. Tried and tested. Back in the old days they even had a cabbage soup recipe that you could make and eat all you wanted. (As if *that* would fill the empty spaces like chocolate would.)

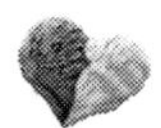

Over the years I encountered some bizarre diets. I remember one in particular, supposedly designed for cardiac patients who had to lose weight quickly before they could have heart surgery. The first day you could eat all the fruit you wanted. Second day, all the veggies you wanted but nothing else. Third day was all fruits and vegetables. Your big reward at the end of that day was to be allowed to have a huge baked potato, with butter. The rest of the week included skim milk and brown rice, some lean meat, and God knows what else! It would be hard to get through even two days on that one!

Then I watched some of my friends go on an extreme diet that involved getting daily injections of some magic drug or other, plus cutting their calories to 500 per day. They were often bragging how much weight they'd lost in a very short time. I was thinking, duh, anyone who cuts their calories back to 500 per day (just short of starving) would lose substantially, with or without the damned injections! Count me out!

In fact, every time I decided to lose weight my next step was to run to Dairy Queen to get myself a "last supper" Blizzard. After that I'd hit the grocery store for my favorite can of mixed gourmet nuts. Then I'd run home and make up a batch of brownies and gulp them all down that same night, since on most diets I'd not be seeing any of these foods for a long, long time to come. The usual result was that I'd generally *gain* five pounds in the first 24 hours of the diet!

I confess I'm a closet junk food junkie. A choco-holic. A sugar addict. Whatever terminology you want to use. And while I understand that America's obesity epidemic is at an all time high, whenever I go to my doctor's office and they give me the usual paperwork to fill out, they're (thankfully) more worried about my other behaviors. They always ask if I smoke and how much. Or if I drink and how much. Or even if I do drugs, to which I always wonder just how many people lie about this. They even ask me if I have any sexual problems, to which I usually reply, "Does not having someone who wants to be intimate regularly with me constitute a problem?" They rarely get the joke. But I ask you, if obesity is such a huge thing then why aren't they asking us about it right along with the drugs, alcohol, or tobacco? Or do they just zero in on what the scales shouts the minute they make you step on it? I wonder.

I should clarify my eating habits just a bit. Sure, I eat salads and meats and veggies – sometimes. But mostly I eat every unhealthy food out there and, quite frankly, I don't want to give it up. *But*, I don't want to carry around unnecessary weight either. I literally want to have my cake and eat it too! Doesn't everyone?

This is my journey to do just that. I call this book a dieter's memoir that reads like a novel (and a self-help book) but with a twist, and it's a big one: Incredibly, I discovered that I really can eat anything I want and still lose weight. Even my dog reshaped her girlish figure right along with me. Neither she nor I saw that coming!

But it was a bumpy road.

This is my true story, my 40-year journey that taught me there is No Cheatin' – Just Eatin'.

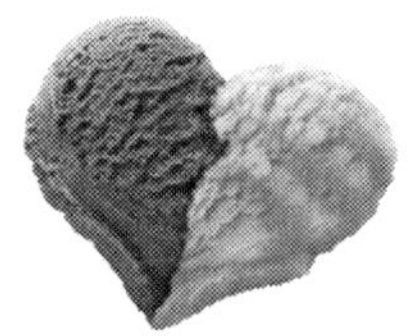

CHAPTER 2

But I'm Not That Bad – Am I?

My story starts with a mirror. I often wondered if it could possibly be one of those at the circus in the house of mirrors. The kind that made you fatter than you really were. I could hope, couldn't I?

Here I was, for the zillionth time again sadly staring at my naked body reflecting back at me from the full-length mirror in my bedroom. My little, white Schnauzer, Larkin, curled up at the foot of my bed, was watching stoically.

"What do you think, girl?" I asked.

I kept hoping she'd say something encouraging as a girlfriend would, like, "What are you talking about? You look great," or at least, "Not to worry ... your weight's not *that* bad." I'd been trying to teach her English for more than four years and she just wasn't getting it. She yawned and then began licking her crotch instead. Obviously more important to her. She had issues too, after all.

Returning to my nakedness, I looked back at my reflection with my harsh critical eye and groaned, as usual. At 5'8" and 175 pounds I certainly wasn't morbidly obese. But my body felt like it was rebelling against me these days. I'd certainly weighed much less at many different times in my life. And not just all the way back in high school.

Staring straight at myself, I began the painful judgment routine, starting with my arms, which I have to confess, weren't too bad. I posed like Popeye, lifting each bent arm towards the sky and was pleased to see a couple of muscle definitions there. At least all the time spent at the gym doing arm workouts was accomplishing something. So, OK, the arms weren't bad.

I moved down to my breasts. Yes, I could even tolerate them, for the most part – ironically, after many years of hating them. God had simply been way too generous with me in that department. As an athlete in high school and an equestrienne for years, too much boob was simply too much boob! For those who need further explanation, try strapping two heavy water balloons to your chest, then go jogging or, even worse, gallop full tilt on a fiery steed. Not pretty. And certainly not comfortable.

Then there were the comments that came and, even worse – *the looks*, from the males of the species. It always seemed to me that they thought we women ordered boobs in whatever size we wanted and, if a gal was pretty chesty, she obviously had ordered boobs in a larger size because she was looking to *use* them somehow. And when that was the case, the looks were even more obnoxious.

Those secretive looks were one thing. The slobbering, put-your-tongue-back-in-your-mouth looks were about as pathetic and embarrassing as you could get. What made it worse were the guys who never could connect with a girl's eyes but could only stare her in the chest. My daughter used

 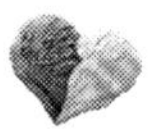

to talk about that phenomenon in high school and how she and her friends had come up with a defense against the look. Their response was, "You might as well look up here," (pointing to their eyes) "because you're not going to be meeting these girls anytime soon!"

I remember staying over at a college boyfriend's house one night, when I hadn't planned to do so, and as such, had no PJ's of my own. He lent me one of his T shirts and as I pulled it over my head and settled the girls comfortably in place he turned to me and said, "Looks like a couple of rabbits fighting for air in a sack in there!" Need I say more? That memory is burned in my brain in intimate detail.

Then there was the time when I was on the girl's track team in high school. One day, we were out jogging around the track warming up while the boys were still fooling around, waiting for their coach to arrive. As the girls' team jogged by, smiling and flirting with all those cute boys in their cute little gym shorts (think 1974, before big, baggie shorts took over), the boys all picked up the chant of, "Bounce, bounce, bounce," as the girls and their entertaining breasts bounced by.

Well, their comments raised quite a stir with the girls' parents, so next time we bounced our way past the boys, their new chant was, "No derogatory remarks, no derogatory remarks!" Which only changed the verbiage but not the meaning.

I also remember one day walking across the street in my little hometown of 12,000 people, three stoplights and one Hardee's. It was much like Mayberry. People were generally decent. And yet, there were still jerks among them.

It was summer. I was crossing the street in the middle of the two-block downtown. I was wearing a T-shirt. The girls were tucked neatly in a nice, supportive bra. Suddenly a man slowed his car and stopped, then waved me across at the crosswalk. Then, just as I got near his front bumper, he yelled out, "Nice set of lungs you got there, Sister."

As a naive 18 year old, I really didn't know what to do with that. All I can tell you is that to this day I avoid wearing T shirts at all cost.

That was yet one more example of how the male of the species seemed to think we order our boobs in the size suited to our intention. Of course in today's world of widespread breast augmentation, that assumption is more true than untrue but it certainly wasn't the case in 1974.

I was, however, especially pleased that I'd undergone a breast reduction when I was about 30, despite my husband's objection. Bringing the girls into a more reasonable size. Yet, at present, as I gaze into that mirror, they have crept back up to 40-D's with a bit more droop than I was hoping for, but gravity does have its way over the years. At least a good bra generally holds them in fairly well, with substantial cleavage that will catch the male of the species' eye at least. So the boobs, all in all, I could live with them.

But, as I moved farther south as I looked in that mirror, I ran into my nemesis – my God-awful belly. My critical eyes immediately went to my poochy tummy that made me look about five months pregnant, especially when I turned the view to profile. (I turned it profile then, just to prove the point.) Ugh. It was still there.

I'd only had one child, for God's sake. Only one. How could only one innocent baby leave me with such a pooch? And years ago, to boot. I didn't even have any stretch marks!

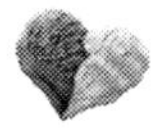

And I'd only gained 13 pounds when I was pregnant, as I'd spent the first four or five months puking my guts out. In fact, the day after I delivered my daughter and went to the nursery to get her to go home, the discharge nurse who had not seen me before, looked questioningly at me as I didn't look like the other new moms, whose tummies still looked pregnant. After all, between the months of puking as well as teaching an aerobics class until I was seven months pregnant, my body was in pretty good shape.

Even better still was when I jumped on the scale at the nurse's station and was shocked at what I saw. I asked, "Is this thing accurate?" The nurse replied, "Yes, it is. All the new moms hate it and swear it can't be right. Not to worry, though. You'll lose your baby weight real soon."

What she didn't know was that I weighed 150 pounds that day after I gave birth, which was the same amount I weighed when I conceived! While all the other moms were lamenting the battles they faced getting their girlish figures back, my weight was already gone.

What the heck happened to that cooperative belly from my baby-bearing year, I wanted to know?

It seems, these days, that any extra weight I added took a bee-line for the gut. "Belly fat," as it is commonly referred to today. All the magazines and books are reminding us that belly fat is the most dangerous for our health, and the hardest to get rid of once it sets up housekeeping in your body.

I sucked my gut in as I always did during these naked body checks, holding my breath. Yep, if I could just drop those damned 20 extra pounds that the scale was pleased to inform me of – and, if it all could come off directly from my belly – I knew I would feel so much better about myself.

Here I was, staring at my pooch again. And it didn't just haunt me when I was naked either. It caught my attention every time I went to slip into clothes that had a zipper or a button at my waist. Not to mention something as torturous as panty hose! Oh my God. Talk about feeling miserable. I gave up wearing those years ago and if I absolutely had to wear some kind of stockings, I would wear thigh highs and thanked my lucky stars for whoever invented them.

I returned to my critique. One last look, with only the butt and the legs to go. Since I was still on the sideways view, I was pleased to see that I was still keeping the cellulite at bay there and, in fact, even had some muscle definition on each side, which had to be the result of years of staying busy, athletically. My calves were OK too. At least no complaints there. Whew.

I guess I liked my legs the best. At least until 2011 when I had both my knees replaced due to the disappearance of all cartilage in both of them with resultant, constant pain. (The downside to a lifetime of major physical activity – for me, anyway.) The scars had softened somewhat over time, but still looked like someone had taken a white piece of chalk and drawn an 8-inch line down both knee caps, heading towards my toes.

Thank God they weren't any worse than that – I'd seen some other folks' scars and some weren't as pretty as mine. And while I was glad my state of affairs wasn't any worse than it was, I did miss my pretty knees of a younger age. However, I was much happier with working knees, I have to admit. I didn't miss the pain either. And the fact that they still got me around fairly well, I couldn't complain too much.

One last check; I grabbed my hand mirror and turned my back to the floor-length mirror to study the rear view –

 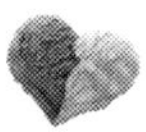

already knowing what I'd find there. I smiled. My butt and I had had a fair relationship over the years. While it was a bit flat, it wasn't horrible to look at. Cellulite didn't seem to hide there. Years of horse-back riding must have pounded it in shape, I guess. I could live with it. It wouldn't win any body-builder competitions, but it did OK in a skirt.

But all the parts of my body that were not so bad didn't stand a chance of being noticed over that damn belly. It haunted me. It felt like it called me names every single day. I hated the muffin top that showed up in most of my clothes. And on top of that, add any little indigestion or bloating and forget buttoning anything. And those days of two-piece bathing suits only a handful of years ago; well, I wasn't in any rush to return *there*.

As to the rest of my wardrobe, most of my clothes were size 14 but some of them weren't too comfy anymore either. I absolutely drew the line at buying anything size 16. But I could sense that line was already growing pretty shaky.

I stuck out my tongue at the reflection, as I frequently did. And after slipping into my sweats, I headed to the kitchen to find something sweet to fill the empty space within me that either couldn't accept myself the way I was, or wouldn't give myself the firm kick in the butt that I needed to do something different.

I've rarely been totally and completely happy with my body, but for the most part, it has served me well. While I have never been obese, and have been pretty physically active most of my life, most people don't realize that I generally do battle with my weight, maxing out at 196 pounds a few years back. Now *that* was scary. And seeing just how close the number

200 was each time I got on the scale left me terrified. This was a boundary I MUST NOT BREAK!

I liken the cause of my binging times (and any time I seem to balloon up) to something overwhelming like depression, which comes and goes with various issues in my life – like no-man-in-my-life times, for one.

Funny how, whenever I gain weight and it shows in the fact that my clothes don't fit anymore, I subtly move from jeans to leggings, stretchy yoga pants, or shorts so I don't have to worry about fit or comfort. At the same time I realize that not worrying about those issues allows me to actually compound the problem by providing even more built-in space to accommodate more fat! Vicious cycle.

This revelation occurred to me at one point, during my heaviest of times, when a neighbor asked me why she had never seen me in jeans. Did I even own any? *Of course*, I thought. Way in the back of my closet for those hopeful times that I might fit into them again.

Ironically, the same neighbor who pointed this oddity out to me indeed wore jeans, despite being substantially overweight herself. Of course, I'm not sure she'd have looked better in leggings, had she tried that option. Her thighs were her enemy. In her case, the right-size, roomy jeans seemed to be the smartest move. Yet for me, the idea of handing over more money for yet a larger, roomier pair of jeans to live quietly in my closet unworn during another weight gain, just didn't sit well. I stuck with the leggings and stretchy things for the time being. Thinking I was fooling myself, but not.

For the last couple of years I'd been stuck at 175 pounds, which for someone my height is approximately 20 pounds too much. But that was after losing 40 and then gaining 20 back.

 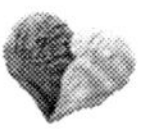

While I realize that I'm not in high school anymore, I do remember weighing about 148 pounds while on the track team and being about as fit as I could ever get. So, considering I'm no longer a hormonal, high energy teen who burns weight even while asleep, I'm comfy compromising my ideal weight to sit right around 155. I was last there (for a relatively short time) in 2009 when I managed to drop 30 pounds before my daughter's wedding. (Great incentive, right?) I then dropped 10 more after that, over the next few months.

God, I loved that time when my body felt just wonderful and I couldn't wait to pull on my skinny jeans! Of course I was also almost an addict to my weight loss at that time. In fact during the race to be skinny for all those wedding photos I was not only counting every calorie that went in my mouth, I was also working out twice per day! And included in those workouts was running about 40 miles per week! Get my drift regarding the addiction part?

So, you might be wondering, if I lost 40 pounds once, why couldn't I simply lose 20 now? Why didn't I just do what I'd done before?

Ah, that's where I get ahead of myself. It all actually started one summer day in 1975 ...

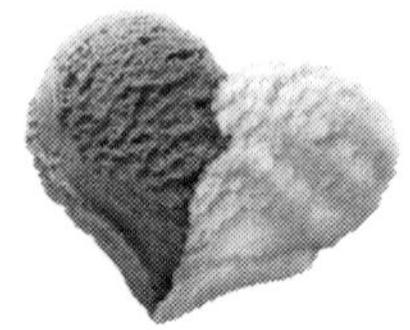

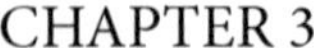

CHAPTER 3

"My God Girl, Have You Gotten Fat!"

I grew up in tiny, little Whitewater, Wisconsin; population 12,000 with a small state university, and lots and lots of farming and milk cows. It was also so small that everyone knew everyone's business. And as for us kids, we never got away with anything as our parents had a network of spies keeping track of our every move. Who needed security cameras back then? You want an example?

I remember walking home from school one day as a high schooler. Normally I would have taken the bus but it was a beautiful day and I had a hankering to stop and buy a brownie at the local bakery on my way home. After indulging myself in the heaven-sent chocolate, I headed the rest of the way home and as I opened the door my mom greeted me with, "So, I hear you stopped at the bakery on the way home!" *Caught!* I felt like I was stalked by the CIA or something. I never tried smoking or drinking or God forbid, pot for fear that one of my mom's spies would have reported back to her before I'd have even gotten started.

 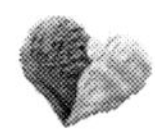

Just one of the joys of living in a small town!

Of course the parents loved it, since it was hard for kids to even think about getting into trouble to begin with. And any stranger in town came under instant scrutiny as a potential danger. I have to say, I always felt safe living there with that tight network in place.

Yet the other side of the small-town coin was the gossip. Gossip about everyone and everything was just a part of life as well. With no cable TV or Internet yet, the daily goings-on was front page news on the weekly paper, the *Whitewater Register*. Who did this and who did that was more important sometimes than Walter Cronkite's news.

My mom's favorite expression was, "What would the neighbors say?" Which guided any and all behaviors. As if the neighbor's and everyone else's opinions mattered more than our own.

Of course there were bullies back then too. And one day, a few years later, I ran into one completely by accident and it changed my life, and my relationship with food, forever. (Although I didn't know it at the time.) It took place, believe it or not, at the one and only 7-Eleven store in town ...

* * *

I had headed into the 7-Eleven on a mission. In reality, being the junk food junkie I was, even back then, I was on a quest to get my next fix, which at that moment consisted of two Hostess Cupcakes and a Reese's Peanut Butter Cup.

Yes, all for me. And double yes – all for me right now.

I paid the red-headed, bored-looking teenage girl behind the counter for my treasures and headed towards the door, salivating the entire way. Paying heed to no one. I was so focused that I didn't even see anyone else in the store once the clerk took my money. I was 100% zeroed in on achieving that euphoria from the high fructose corn syrup, artificially sweetened, Red Dye #2, loaded with preservative yummies that I knew would leave me feeling quite happily buzzed for the rest of the next few hours, anyway.

My taste buds were on high alert, counting the seconds it would take until I could frantically tear off the cellophane wrapper and dive in head-first to get that incredible rush; not only from the luscious cupcakes but also from that amazing smell of the Reese's Peanut Butter Cups. Decisions, decisions. Which one should I eat first? As always, I chose the one that opened the easiest. There's nothing more frustrating that needing your sugar fix and the damned package won't open. You want to talk about panic attack?

I've never done drugs – not even pot – but I am convinced that my addiction to sweets was probably just as emotionally messed up as if I were a cocaine addict. I just didn't want to wait one more second to feel my teeth sink into that dark, yummy confection, never mind that it had enough preservatives to keep it edible for the next 50 years. I didn't care a lick what was in it. I just ached to feel it on my tongue, on my teeth, in my blood stream and as soon as possible. My heart rate was already beginning to increase as my mind sent it messages of anticipation.

And so, my conscious mind barely heard the words that rang out next – it was too busy anticipating the first burst of flavor of the delectable goody on my tongue. But my subconscious mind must have been paying some attention because I

 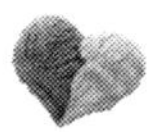

found myself stopped dead in my tracks, freezing in the spot as I heard someone say, in a good strong voice, "My God, girl, have you gotten fat!"

Whoa! Who, I wondered, was the bully that was speaking so inappropriately? And who was the poor sucker who was being judged and belittled in such a horrid way? My eyes quickly scanned the 7-Eleven for possible candidates, as I'd not really paid attention to anyone or anything else during the acquisition of my fix. The cupcake had 110% of my attention 'til then.

Glancing around, I ruled out the red-headed teenager who had waited on me. She couldn't have been more than five feet tall and skinny as a lot of girls are while still in their teens. There was an older Latino couple studying the menu at the fast food corner where hot dogs, that looked like they'd been there all day, were slowly grilling on the rotating wiener roaster. But both husband and wife were busy in their own little world. Neither of them were what I would consider fat, anyway.

A tall, brunette mom in her 20's with a new baby in her arms looked to be pretty fit, so no, it was likely not her, although she had every right to be so, having given birth only recently, by the looks of things.

Having studied all the options, I was stumped. Who was the alleged fat girl and who was the mean playground bully? And then I realized that as I had been opening the door to head out, someone else had been opening the other side of the door on her way in. And that someone looked familiar. Really familiar. But I just couldn't place who she might be. If I could only get my mind off the damned cupcake for long enough to put 2 and 2 together, I might figure out just who had thrown the jab at, oh my God, ME!

"Geeze, MJ," came the voice again, "I almost didn't recognize you, you've gotten so fat!" she repeated. She wasn't much older than me, I realized. And was *really* tall – taller than me actually. Nearly 6 feet as I recall. She had long, straight, dirty blonde hair and wore tortoise shell glasses that made her look like a college professor or maybe a librarian. I realized that she had an expression that was demanding an explanation of some sort. And she gave me the impression that she would likely not move until I gave her one.

My mind kept racing. She obviously knew me, since she called me by name. I searched my memory banks for ID recognition but my damned sugar high just kept clouding everything. Then, suddenly there was a stabbing pain in my chest and abdomen. I realized that I had started hyperventilating – or at least it felt like that must be what was happening based on all the medical shows I'd watched on TV. I kid you not. I couldn't breathe. Not realizing it at the time, my body was tuning in to the old "fight or flight" response, which obviously wasn't doing too well up to that point because I wasn't able to flee. And, if I couldn't breathe soon, the odds are I'd pass out and likely hit the floor.

My mind reached for those scathing words again ... What did she say? Me? Fat? I have NEVER been fat. There must be some mistake. Why on Earth would anyone say that? It must be some stupid joke.

The sharp pain in my abdomen continued but a new symptom joined the foray – my face began to turn bright red, along with one ear. I could feel it! What the hell was happening to me? It seemed like I was having one of my mother's hot flashes that left her acting like a crazy person, racing back and

 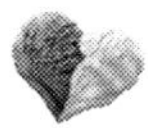

forth to the freezer every few minutes to get ice for her ice pack or cool off next to the open freezer door. But I was way too young for that. In theory, I was too young to have a heart attack as well. And yet my symptoms were classic – for a 40 year old!

The internal volcano of heat caused by what I later realized was overwhelming embarrassment is what I could feel had lit up my face like a second-degree sunburn. I think today they call it a panic attack. But at that moment, I didn't know what the hell it was. I just knew that it left me terrified. And frozen in space and time. On top of that, try as I might, I couldn't utter a single word or even breathe through my mouth. Which wasn't just because I'd felt like my life as I knew it might just fall apart at any moment. The real reason I couldn't reply was that only seconds earlier I had stuffed a giant bite of a Hostess cupcake in my face and now it was stuck there.

You'd think I could have at least waited to eat the damned thing in private or taken it home to devour. But no – as soon as I'd swapped coins for the cupcake with the kid behind the counter, I couldn't wait to rip open the cellophane wrapper.

My mind had been picturing me devouring that delectable delight for about 30 minutes before I had even arrived at the store. Once there, true to form, I had taken a huge bite before I headed out. That's one of those crazy addictive behaviors I have to admit to being embarrassed about. And now I was caught.

Then I started coughing as I tried to say something to this woman, but the damned cupcake was still stuck in my throat. That only made things worse. In the end, I pantomimed to the unrecognized gal with my free hand that I really couldn't stay and chat. Had to go. Catch you later. Then raced to my car, threw in my stash, leapt in and sped out of the parking lot, praying that no one else would see me that day, or possibly ever.

I remember that I could barely see the road through my tears. I was still in shock. I never considered *myself* fat. In fact I remember when I was about 12 or so telling everyone that I was so skinny that my jeans kept falling off. And that was kinda my self-image for years. Skinny MJ who never had to worry about what I ate. Of course as a 12 year old I hadn't considered that most of my jeans I inherited from a cousin who was a couple of years older than me and between the time she'd outgrown them and the time they actually fit me as they should, they indeed were often falling off if I didn't have a belt. They were just too big!

Honestly, I am not making this up. I was thin most of my young life. At least I *thought* I was up until that day. I hadn't yet been taunted by the negative little voice in my head that criticized me if I didn't do something right. That little devil voice would come later. As a naive 12 year old I still had all my Mojo; the happy little voice in my head that said I could do or be whoever or whatever I wanted to be. That I had all the ability and talents I needed to do absolutely anything. That I was a wonderful and amazing person just as I was.

You know the voice; you have one too. We all do. You may not have a name for it. I didn't at the beginning. She was just my gutsiness, the cheerleader in my head, my mojo. Sometimes she was there when I needed her and sometimes she laid low, awaiting my decisions, then cheering me on when I made the right ones. Over time, as we grew closer, she became my Miss Mojo.

 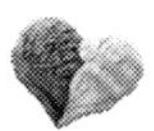

But that day even Miss Mojo was knocked off guard and had no idea how to fix this.

I was lucky to make the drive home without running into anything or anyone, at the same time still stuffing my goodies in my mouth, trying to fill the hole, the wound, the anguish I'd been through. I immediately went to the mirror and tried to see myself through my tear-filled eyes. Funny, I still felt like the same person – the one who was OK with herself prior to the event. But I felt I needed a reassessment of the image that the world saw when they looked at me ...

To start with, my very short, blonde hair always made me stand out from the crowd. I remember seeing that style on the cover of a *Seventeen* magazine right before my high school graduation. I thought it was soooo cool! So much so that the day after I graduated from high school, and without warning anyone I was going to do this, I went to the beauty shop and had them cut my shoulder-length locks into this totally rebellious Audrey Hepburn/Mia Farrow look. My mother about flipped when I walked in the front door, with my new look. Unannounced. I actually thought for a moment she might pass out. I'm pretty sure she never forgave me, since she never ceased to retell this story over the years. Far from what most of the other college girls wore, and not with any lesbian presumptions at a time when *that* hadn't even come on the scene yet, I felt it gave me a unique look. I think that maybe I was trying to assert my independence with that short haircut. Maybe. Probably.

However, most fads like that run their course and soon *Seventeen* magazine featured something else new and different on their covers, leading the fashions in whatever direction was in favor at the time, but I never grew my hair long again. While there were mild deviations of it over the years, it's rather become my brand. And all because I wanted to be a bit defiant in 1975!

Anyway, back to my critical mirror assessment ... so here I was at 5'8". No hiding that. I rather liked being tall, especially since I towered over all the women in my family. Although the opposite side of that is that I oftentimes felt gangly. Can you say, "Jolly Green Giant"? I was taller than most of the boys, and that wasn't necessarily so great.

My piercing hazel eyes (many would insist they were blue over the years but I still saw the green and grayish hues in them that would show up from time to time) captivated many. In fact, a lot of people commented on them and still do. An optometrist once told me I should be an eye model. Which was cool since I still thought they just looked like plain, ordinary eyes to me.

Then there was my *fashion statement*. My style. My college freshman look. Back in 1976 the hippy, college student, rebellious version of fashion found me wearing my old standby: a pair of slightly faded farmer's overalls – the kind with the adjustable hooks over each collar bone and a couple of buttons down near the hips, which could also be treated as optional, in case growing room was needed. Throw a baggy t-shirt or sweatshirt under that and a pair of tennies (they still called them that back then) and my outfit was complete. What was wrong with that?

Little did I realize that while they were all the rage for the day and oh-so comfy, those nasty bugger overalls did me no favors. I could have probably packed on an extra 50 pounds

 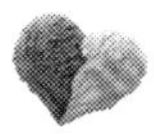

and my overalls would have done a great job of making more room. There is no button at your middle to button up when you're wearing these "designer" items, as there is with regular blue jeans. But with overalls: Need more room? Just unbutton those optional buttons at the waist and they'll be glad to make more room. The truth of the matter is, I simply hadn't noticed the daily gain because those baggy overalls just kept finding room for me! Or, at least, that's my story.

On top of that, I didn't have a bathroom scale in my apartment, so I only checked my actual weight on occasion when I stopped by my parents' home or at the gym for some PE class or other. I guess I must not have had any kind of weight chart that I remember either, so just kept eating myself silly without even recognizing it. Until that day at the 7-Eleven.

Well, I never forgot those few poignant words. I did finally remember the gal from 1975 who had felt the need to turn my world upside down with her scalding remarks. It was Kathy, and I had gone to high school with her, although she was two years older than me and had gone to college out of state, so I hadn't seen her in a long time. Obviously long enough that I'd had time to pack on the pounds during my freshman year at college and she felt the need to tell me about it.

Looking back at it now, I realize that she was talking about my obvious Freshman 15, although at that point it was more like the Freshman 30, if I'm being honest with myself. But there-in lies the rub – I WASN'T being honest with myself. In fact I was in complete denial. I'd always been thin but had never lived the life of a college freshman and the hazards that often go along with the role. I truly had no realization that in one year's time I had really packed on the pounds.

A couple of ironies, however, about Kathy and me. She wasn't anything to write home about. She had always been about 25-30 pounds overweight herself and not particularly talented physically. That is, she was the last one picked for any game in PE class, always. Whereas I had always been busy with athletics; I ran the mile in track back when no girls wanted to run that far! I was on the volleyball team when girls volleyball was just getting organized at the high school level. I even played slow-pitched softball on a city league. I biked, swam, and rode horses whenever I could talk my neighbor or uncle into letting me ride theirs.

For the first 18 years of my life I never had to think twice about what I ate. I just ate it! No matter what "it" was. And never felt guilty about it either. Never even had that nagging, little devil voice in my head yet, saying I was bad for downing 3 or 4 cookies instead of the 2 everyone else had at school.

Ah, yes! Those were the days!

So much happened between those days and the day that Kathy knocked me off my pedestal at the 7-Eleven. (By the way, I don't think she was really intending to be mean, I think she was just in total shock about how much my body had changed.)

And yet, who was she to talk? I wondered. Her body was nothing to write home about. In fact, I wouldn't be surprised if she'd put on another 20 pounds on top of what she already carried since I'd seen her last. I hated her for a long time for sending me home in tears that day, and for the hurtful memories that have lasted all these years.

However, I thank her now for being the only person willing to tell me the truth about my body when no one else would.

 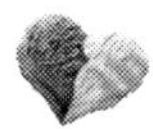

I shudder to think if no one would have called me on my weight gain, and I had gained even more. I still don't know if it's smart to tell your family member or friend that they have a weight problem, but if you are going to do so, hopefully it will be in a much nicer way than Kathy did. But still, it's a tricky spot to be in. One usually assumes that a heavy person knows that they are heavy. But in my situation, I was in major denial until her words came crashing down on me. In my mind, I just didn't feel "that bad."

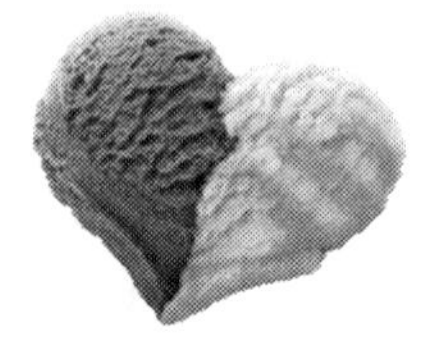

CHAPTER 4

A Playboy Bunny Or A Cowgirl?

I lost weight that first time, not by dieting, but by working it off. Not long after the 7-Eleven incident I became a cowgirl. Certainly not something I ever anticipated, but definitely effective. But I'm getting a bit ahead of myself again.

I had been a horse-crazy kid for as long as I could remember, and when my elderly neighbor, Mr. Jackson, bought a pony for his grandkids when I was in the 5th grade, I felt like I'd died and gone to heaven. He named her Queenie. She was a little Shetland pony, mostly white with a few reddish patches and a rogue mane and tail that always looked like she was having a bad hair day – despite my friend Denise and I brushing and doting over her for hours nearly every day. Mr. Jackson gave us carte blanche with her and as my dad had worked with horses on the farm where he grew up, he was able to teach us to ride.

We got to be pretty good, actually. In part, because Queenie had no saddle, only a bridle. So, we learned to ride bare back and developed good balance from the get-go. You either learned to hold on tight with your legs or else you'd hit the ground. The very hard ground. Once we became pretty good

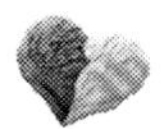

at it, there was one more challenge: Queenie was quirky. You had to play by her rules. If you wanted her to canter, you had to slap her with her long reins on her behind and she would buck once, then pick up the pace to a steady, comfortable little gallop. If you could hang in there long enough to get through the buck, it was smooth sailing.

I was fortunate to learn a few facts of life from Queenie too – when Mr. Jackson brought another pony named Moses to "visit … for a few weeks" as he put it. Eleven months later, right as Denise and I were doing our daily doting on what we felt was "our" pony (the grandkids never did want to ride), Queenie gave birth right in front of us to a darling little boy they named Prince. He was opposite in color to his mom – mostly red with a few splotches of white here and there. Denise and I were true believers in God at that point. We had carte blanche with two ponies that could well have been our own, for all the time we spent with them.

Unfortunately, God had different plans for Mr. Jackson, and called him up to heaven about the time Prince was a year old, which definitely wrecked our world. Mrs. Jackson sold the farm and packed up to move to the city, but not before she told me I could keep Prince if it was OK with my parents.

Thank you, Jesus. There was a God, I was more certain than ever. My world had just been saved...

...Until my parents put pen to paper, as they put it, and started adding up just what it costs to keep a pony – especially when we didn't own any land to keep it on. It didn't take a mathematician to figure out that horses are expensive – even in small size. Plus there were four kids in my family. Four mouths to feed. And how would it be fair if I got a pony and none of the others did? (Not that any of them wanted one! And besides, the other three kids were already out of the house!) Sadly, Mom and Dad's answer was a resounding, "No."

Explaining the financial facts of life to an 11 year old in love with a couple of ponies did not go well. I think I cried for a week. And I think it was closer to several years before I forgave them.

Fortunately I had an uncle who had a couple of horses I could bum a ride off of, from time to time, and my dad would occasionally take me to a nearby livery stable for my horse fix. While it wasn't the same as the days of wine and ponies, I did learn to be a pretty good rider over the years.

...Which started me on the path to becoming a cowgirl. Or maybe more appropriately, a wrangler.

My first job with horses was in Lake Geneva, Wisconsin in 1974 at a facility that today is called the Grand Geneva, but at that time was the Playboy Club Hotel. No, I was NOT a bunny, although back then I was still overly endowed and, as such, (and working at such a facility to begin with,) led many to think I was, despite lacking a traditional bunny suit. I guess my boots and jeans didn't make it clear that I was a horsie gal, not a bunny gal! Once again, men seemed to think that we ladies chose what size boobs we had for a reason and that we chesty gals were meant to be ogled. And ogle they did.

I took folks on trail rides around the beautiful grounds hailing two full-sized golf courses, a gorgeous lake, and a very modern-looking, sprawly hotel. Mostly Chicago people would venture up to the tourist town over the weekends. And they came in droves. Some days were so busy at the stables that we didn't eat all day. And my Freshmen 30 started to pare down

 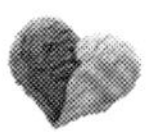

rather painlessly. I still had my addiction, and could always grab one of my favorite Hostess goodies that my mom kept around for my sack lunches. Did I mention I loved the pies as well?

The guy who ran the stables did not work for the hotel itself. The stables were a concession and he was the manager. And a horrible one at that. He penny-pinched wherever he could, including adding very expired bread and pastries to the horses' feed. He apparently thought that, since bread was made out of grains and, since horses ate grain, why wouldn't they want to eat pastries? Plus, many of the delicacies were covered in sweet, sugary drizzled frosting. So, therefore, if horses liked sugar cubes, they'd love frosting. And they did! He got the week-old stuff for next to nothin' at a local bakery and was quite pleased with himself for finding yet another way to shave his expenses – whether it was good for the horses or not.

I have to admit it was funny watching them inhale hot dog and hamburger buns, coffee cake, and loaves of bread. Sometimes they looked like they were smoking big Cuban cigars when a hot dog bun would be part way in and part way out of their mouths. To me, it was just wrong in so many ways.

I only bring this up because a funny thing happened one day while we wrangler kids actually had a slow day, with time for lunch for a change, and someone had run out for fast food. We were sitting on a bench devouring our burgers from the local A & W, chatting away. To my back was a very large stall that held the two, huge draft horses that pulled the hay wagon – another one of those touristy items every stable has.

I had been working on my burger and chatting in between bites, gesturing with my right hand, which was holding the still-warm sandwich, when suddenly, out of nowhere, poof! It disappeared.

I blinked my eyes, in an attempt to re-focus the burger back into sight, but couldn't. I was totally confused. Then one of my fellow wranglers started laughing his butt off as he'd watched the scene take place. One of the big draft horses, one who obviously was a fan of the bakery fare, had promptly grabbed my sandwich from my gesturing hand and inhaled it in one gulp into his gigantic mouth! He wolfed it down greedily in a few chomp-chomps with his equally enormous teeth – before most of us knew what had happened! Then he started eyeing the others' lunches as well, hopeful that another one might wander by his stall, as unsuspecting as I had been.

We all laughed ourselves silly over that one and, in the future, guarded our personal foods (my Hostess goodies, for sure) from the greedy equines! That was a pretty fun summer and set the groundwork for more serious cowboy-in and working my weight off.

* * *

It was mid May, 1976 and I was on a tiny plane flying from Denver International Airport to Granby, Colorado, about 60 miles west of Denver, high up in the mountains at nearly 8,000 feet. I had been hired as a wrangler for the C-Lazy-U Dude and Guest Ranch and I was scared to death. Not about the job ... I was super excited about the job. But I'd only flown twice before and that had been on a big commercial air liner to Washington, D.C. the previous summer and then the flight that had just brought me to Denver. Those were

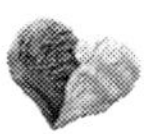

pretty scary as it was, for a newbie flyer such as myself, but it got worse. The little hopper plane held about 20 folks and with the turbulence in the mountain air that day, the damned thing was bouncing all over the place and the oxygen masks had fallen from their little spaces over each seat and some people actually were using them.

I didn't know what I was supposed to do. No one seemed to be upset besides me. I figured out later that most of the passengers were regulars to the situation and had gotten pretty used to the little plane in the rough currents – thus their lack of apparent fear. I think I must have prayed for the entire 30-minute flight and by the time we landed I was an emotional wreck.

As the little plane landed at the Granby airport I was surprised yet again ... the terminal was about the size of a small house trailer with room to hold a handful of people. I hadn't known what to expect when I booked the ticket. And found out later there were several of these little mountain towns with teeny, tiny airports, mostly for the skier population during the winter.

I'd been worried about my luggage making the transfer from Denver to Granby, and when I climbed out of the plane and watched the luggage guy begin pulling out several suitcases and didn't catch a glimpse of my own, my anxiety began to climb even more. As Luggage Guy emptied the storage compartment and closed the door on it, I was certain my stuff was still in Denver. What was I going to do?

Yet, luck was with me as Luggage Guy opened one more door, exposing several more bags – including mine. I let out a huge sigh of relief. Thank God. Terra Firma and luggage safe. Woo-hoo!

About that time I heard a voice say, "Are you MJ?"

I turned around to see the welcoming face of a handsome young man who looked like he'd been around all of this before. He seemed calm and friendly and polite. His piercing blue eyes sized me up in an instant as a Greenhorn at flying, and I think he only had to try a little bit to keep from chuckling at how I must have looked, as frazzled as I was.

With a huge sigh of relief, I gave a wobbly smile and said, "I love you! Take me away from here!" (How many people have you told you loved them the first time you exchanged words? Not many, I bet.)

I would soon find out that his name was Kevin. Little did I know then that I would marry him two years later.

* * *

The ranch was the only five-star dude ranch in Colorado and Wyoming, and people with lots of money often came for several weeks – to pretend they were cowboys or to just get away from the city. There was a big-shot New York brain surgeon who brought his family to stay for three weeks every summer. Another big-name guest owned an NFL football team. High-powered lawyers and presidents of huge companies were part of the rank and file. There were even people from foreign countries.

The ranch booked 110 guests per week with check-in on Sundays and out on Saturdays. It had been around for years and had such a great reputation that there were never any empty rooms. Activities and amenities included fishing, tennis, golf, skeet and trap shooting, swimming, sauna, dance night, hiking, rafting, and just relaxing with a good book.

 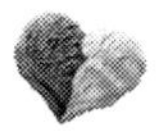

For those who wanted to be a full-time cowboy, they were assigned their own horse for the week. There were even "kiddie counselors" who kept track of all the kids and even the teens and kept them busy and away from their parents from just after breakfast until bedtime each day.

It was an incredible summer, both for my little Mojo voice getting stronger venturing out from my safe, little hometown and dipping my toes into the big, wide world. And getting just about as much horsing around as I could take.

Then of course there was the hormonal factor. With 50 college kids living in such close confinement, sparks were flying all summer long. In fact there were two of us chasing after Kevin for a while. My roommate Holly had her eyes on him too and, for a short while, he was seeing both of us – until we finally smartened up and told him he could have one of us but not both! Suffice it to say, I won.

There were eight of us wranglers – and 110 head of horses that all had to be brushed, grained, and saddled by 9 a.m. six days a week. On top of that, the herd was chased out to pasture every evening, where there were acres and acres of grazing for that many horses. It was quite a sight that the guests loved, as we cowboys and -girls drove the enormous herd down the drive and up to the high pastures in the evenings. The dust they stirred up alone was impressive, and if that coincided with sunset, the waves of moving horse flesh, and with sun's last rays, the sienna color that it produced made everyone feel like they really were back in the old West.

While driving the herd out in the evening was breathtaking, finding all those damned horses again every morning was not so great. Especially for the smartest but laziest of horses who knew enough to hide from us as we hunted them down to go to work. But the old wrangler guy, Don, who had worked there for decades, knew how to outsmart the best of them – especially Big Bertha and her followers, who were pretty good at sizing up just how big a bush they knew to hide behind so as not to be seen.

He'd hang a cowbell over Big Bertha's neck each night before she headed out to the pastures, so whether she was hiding or not, when it was time to be found each morning, if she moved just a few steps we'd hear the bell and could chase her in with the rest of her gang. The horses were pretty funny sometimes. They each had a personality and it was always entertaining to watch their interactions. They were a lot like people in a way. Like Big Bertha, who got sick of the daily grind and tried to get out of work however she could.

More to the point for this story … all the physical work did its magic on me and for once I didn't worry about how much I ate as I wore it off as fast as I inhaled it. Each of those saddles had to weigh twenty-plus pounds and saddling and unsaddling all those horses twice a day outweighed any upper body gym workout you could imagine. Then, there was the all-day poop-scooping after that number of hay burners who turned all that hay into huge, green piles. And lastly, spending four hours in the saddle every day burned up somewhere in the range of 1,200-1,500 calories all on its own. Yep, you really do burn calories riding a horse. By the end of the first month I was fit, fit, fit. And looked amazing in a bikini!

I have to add, there wasn't *time* for me to be snacking all day and night to begin with. And, on top of that, none of us got paid until the end of the first month, so even if I could

 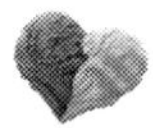

bum a ride into town for a sugar fix with the few kids who actually had a car, I had no extra money to fill up my Hostess wagon.

Things weren't all work and no play at the ranch, however. There were the pranks and the pranksters. Sometimes it was pranks from the regular guests who came every year and who loved to one-up each other with practical jokes and hi-jinks. But sometimes it was the crazy college kids working there who came from all across the country. They would pull all sorts of silly capers on each other as well, just to liven things up a bit.

For an example, the brain surgeon and one of the gals in his group would try to outdo each other – this was an ongoing thing each year. Their tricks included him stealing all her bras and hanging them on the flagpole. She, in turn, filled his bathtub with Jello. He retaliated and put the donkey in her room for an afternoon, which left a pretty nasty smell for quite some time. These pranks continued during their entire stay.

The staff, myself included, had our own tricksters. There was Holly, who one day offered to do Kevin's laundry when she went into town. (He was a manager who rarely got time off to sleep much less do his laundry.) It seems he'd said something that got her upset and she decided to prank him so she hid his laundry for days. (The clean clothes were under his cot the whole time.)

To retaliate, after he recovered his missing laundry, he got his crew together when Holly went into town again. He knocked at my door and said, "MJ, would you mind showing us which bed and which dresser are Holly's, please?"

"Sure," I replied. And I pointed out Holly's furniture. "But what's this all about?" I queried.

"Just a little getting even, that's all," he said, looking guilty as sin. Then he said to his crew, "Boys, you know what to do." And they promptly loaded up and took Holly's stuff out of our room. I hadn't a clue what they were up to, so I followed them. Well, they had perched a ladder on the side of the dorm building and carried Holly's furniture up to the roof! They arranged the furniture on the flat side of the roof, bed neatly made, then came back down the ladder and disappeared.

I'll never forget the look on the faces of a sweet, retired couple from France who had been there all week, who had watched the antics and wondered just how crazy these Americans were out here in the wild West! I had been their interpreter most of the week, as one of the only folks on the ranch who spoke French. And they thought it quite the prank once I explained it to them. They even hung around to await Holly's return.

Well, the reaction was priceless – just as Kevin had hoped. At first glance Holly didn't realize it was her furniture when she saw the scene, and had started laughing when she came down the drive. I don't even think she put 2 and 2 together until she actually came into the dorm and found our room half empty. Then she about had a fit! (It didn't help that some angry storm clouds were moving in! The idea of a soaking wet bed didn't strike her fancy.)

After plenty of begging and pleading, she got someone to help her get her stuff back before it rained. But it was definitely a prank long remembered.

Of course they got me too. And I thought I was pretty lucky with what they did to me – at first. It was the 4th of July

 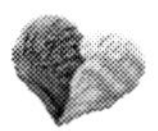

and there was going to be a little parade down the long driveway, with guests and staff alike taking part. I think I'd had to work late that day and so didn't have time to be one of the participants, but was quite happy just to watch all the others in their costumes and convertible cars with their tops down, carrying people dressed up as celebrities of the day. There were people playing instruments, a couple of clowns, someone was leading the burrow, and more.

Then I noticed the next car in line – it carried three young, attractive women, very buxom and animated – sticking out their chests and vigorously waving small American flags. They had sashes that read Miss Colorado, Miss USA, and Miss Universe. They were throwing kisses and flirting with everyone. I wondered who they were. Suddenly I realized that they had the same type of bathing suits that I had ... one piece, brightly colored tanks. One even had an American flag pattern – exactly like mine! Wow! What a coincidence, I naively thought. Then it suddenly occurred to me that those were my bathing suits! And those "girls" were actually three of my co-workers, young men wearing my suits and some very female looking wigs.

They had obviously gotten into my room and snitched the suits while I was working. Where they got the wigs, I never found out. But when they saw me watching, they all turned to me in unison and blew me a big kiss! It was so perfectly timed that they must have practiced this performance as well. Then, they continued along the parade route, flaunting their costumes and their temporary bazooms for all it was worth.

Whew! I thought. If that's all I get pranked with, that was a piece of cake.

But of course, no. That wasn't all. They were still cooking up a much better idea for me, they just hadn't decided exactly what it would be yet. Until a certain mix of circumstances happened that created the perfect opportunity. And I give them credit – it was priceless!

Backing up a bit … to understand how this caper worked you need a couple pieces of the puzzle. Two of the wranglers were vet student guys from New Mexico. The dude ranch wasn't just for dudes – part of its several hundred acres was a real working ranch with real cowboys who kept track of the beef cattle. When one of the calves showed up dead, the vet students insisted on performing an autopsy. Rather, it's called a necropsy when it's an animal. But the story didn't end there.

As I was up at 5 a.m. most mornings and my roommate got to sleep in 'til 6 or so, I would generally turn on the hall light, then open our door to the hallway and get dressed in the bit of light that barely gave me enough brightness to see what clothes I was putting on.

That morning, as I finished pulling on my jeans and shirt, I reached next for my boots, which were the lace-up type work boots. As I picked up the first one and glanced at it, it looked like there was something in it. Since I never kept my socks in my boots, I couldn't figure out what the hell was in there. So, I picked up the boot and took it out into the hallway where I could get full light. And when I did that, my stomach instantly did a 360-degree turn, ready to vomit any second, as I noticed all the blood all over the inside of the boot. I jumped.

"What the hell?!" I hollered, throwing the boot to the ground, not knowing where all that blood had come from. After my heart slowed down from the initial shock, and after

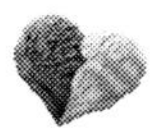

I assured myself that nothing alive was likely going to come out of the boot after me, I picked it up again and rushed into the bathroom/shower area at the end of the hall, where I knew there would be plenty of light and water to help me find out what the hell was at the bottom of this craziness.

As I slowly turned the bloody thing on its side, while positioning myself over the sink, I finally realized what was behind this prank of all pranks – it was the heart of the little calf that the vet students had done the necropsy on!

Jack pot! They sure took the prize for imagination and biggest shock factor! The even bigger impact of the prank was that I only had one pair of boots to my name and, as such, needed to wash them out as best as I could, then put them on and head out to bring in the herd, slimy boot, or no slimy boot! No one ever asked me anything about the boot that morning. We all just acted like nothing mattered. It was kind of the unwritten rule of a prank well done.

I *did* get even, however, although my payback wasn't as awesome as theirs. The guys hit the road for some concert in Denver one night and I knew they'd be getting home very late and would be exhausted and likely just fall into bed. So, to welcome them home I not only short-sheeted their beds but sprinkled Grape Nuts cereal in between their sheets as well – for an extra crispy sleep. I guess they respected my creativity, as no one said a word at breakfast about their nights' sleep. We all just gave each other the look that said, "Well done! Rites of passage, successful!"

I could go on and on with stories from that place but you get the idea. It was definitely a life-changing adventure – and not the last one I would have over the years.

Living away from my folks and my safe, little home town all summer had started to build my confidence and shake off a bit of my naïveté. As I drove down the long driveway for the last time at summer's end, Miss Mojo was strong and confident. And my body was probably in the best shape it had been since my years in high school track.

It couldn't have been a better summer. I had been so happy and, looking back on it now, I realize that whenever I was happy in my life, my weight was never an issue. *That* discovery would prove to be borne out over the years to come. It just took me a long while to realize it.

And, of the 50 college kids who worked there that summer, who also lived through this unique adventure – ten of us would marry each other in the end. How many are still together, I can't say.

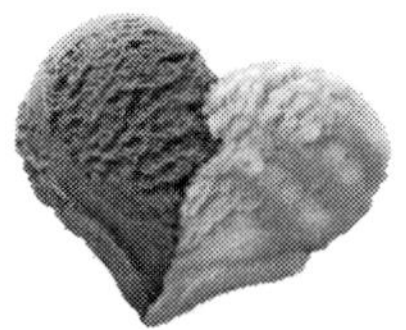

CHAPTER 5

Living The Dream

How the years flew by! So many things happened after that summer that I never could have imagined – both good and bad.

For starters, Kevin and I tied the knot in 1978: two young people in love, with their whole lives ahead of them. As he had already finished college, he moved from Denver to Milwaukee, where I was in nursing school for a couple more years. He took a job as a loan officer for a financial company and I worked part time on the weekends in a movie theatre as a projectionist, back in the days when there was only one movie per theatre. I'd say that's where I got my addiction to movie theatre popcorn, although I never got hooked on the butter flavoring they use. (If you would see what that stuff looks like when it solidifies I guarantee you'd never eat it either!)

As soon as I graduated we packed up our meager belongings and headed back to be close to the mountains that we both loved. We spent countless days hiking the great outdoors together in many of the parks and open spaces that Colorado boasted. And as he'd lived in Denver for many years, it was like having my own, personal forest ranger/guide as well. His family and many of his friends also lived in Denver, so we had a good support network too.

In nursing school I discovered my love of pediatric patients and I really wanted to work for Children's Hospital in Denver. As luck would have it, there was a huge nursing shortage going on then and, by the time I finished my 10 a.m. interview and tour of the hospital, I'd been hired and started orientation class by 1 p.m. My new unit was the Newborn Intensive Care Unit, which at the time, brought us sick, premature, cardiac or surgical newborns from 13 states as there were simply no specialists who could handle those delicate patients out in the boonies of Montana or Wyoming.

As I look back over the years, I loved that kind of nursing the most. We saw everything come in through our doors. And of course sadness as well as they didn't all live. It was quite the education for a young nurse just getting her toes wet in the real world. And spending time with so many young parents in such tough emotional situations helped me develop my own skills of compassion that I would use for the rest of my life.

I'll never forget sitting with one young couple in particular, whose baby was dying. It was their first and she was a perfectly beautiful infant – no one would guess from looking at her that there could possibly be a thing wrong. But she'd been born with an irreparable heart defect and her time on this planet would only be a matter of hours.

We had a private room for families going through these difficult times, and as her nurse, I was available for them, in any way they needed me; close but yet out of their way. They

 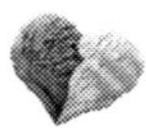

took turns holding their little girl they had named Molly, tears flowing all night. Singing songs to her. Hugging each other. Praying. It was a long night for all of us and by morning the precious little girl had gone with God. By the time the parents gave Molly her last kisses, we'd gone through so much together that they were hugging me too.

I got a letter from them a few days later, thanking me for all my help and remarking what strength I must get from God every day to do my job. Ironically, I didn't have much faith at that time in my life. It would be several years before that blossomed. But the night I spent with that family has remained in my heart all these years.

Over the years I took various other jobs at Children's. One unit I worked on was half kids with infectious diseases and half kids aged 12-ish and younger, with quite a variety of issues. There I learned just how prevalent cleft lips and palates are. And how dangerous brown recluse spider bites are. (The spider's venom had acted like acid on human skin. Very nasty and required skin grafting.) I also helped out on occasion in the burn unit where some very unlucky children had run into some sad circumstances with fire – whether playing with matches to getting caught in house fires, to a toddler pulling a hot iron onto himself, leaving his chest badly scarred forever. I learned first-hand just how painful and destructive fire can be. To this day I rarely have a candle lit in my house.

And the last unit I worked at while at Children's was the pediatric ICU where children with even more complex issues lived or died. From a toddler in Montana who'd been attacked by a wolf, to teens who thought they were invincible and had done stupid things, just goofing off; some that cost them life and limb. There were kids with heart disease who for years had been fighting the good fight with a bleak end in sight, to a couple of girls who'd been in a water skiing accident together. You never knew just what might come in the door. I have to say, it was always exciting. One day I even got to fly in a helicopter with one of the transport nurses, who had to make a run to Vail to pick up a sick kid and they needed an extra hand and asked me if I'd like to go. That was an experience of a lifetime.

But after that first job in the nursery, all the others were in management – still close to the patients but also with supervisory duties. Eventually I became a head nurse for another intensive care nursery in a private general hospital in town where I wore scrubs as my daily uniform.

At the time, I didn't think I had many issues in the weight department. Then I got hit with a moment that brought back the 7-Eleven bad feelings, much to my surprise.

But first, if you've never worn scrubs, let me explain something. Scrubs are worn by surgeons and other medical personnel and look like big baggy sacks over big, baggy pants that close with a drawstring. There is nothing tailored about them. And if you're a Nurse Jackie fan (a show on Netflix) and noticed just how form-fitting Jackie's scrubs are, let me assure you, I've never seen tailored scrubs anywhere besides on that show. I'd even bet you that Edie Falco, (the actress who played Nurse Jackie) had it in her contract that her scrubs would be tailored and slimming. But in real life, they're baggy so they fit just about any body size. While they were comfortable – kinda felt like you were wearing your PJ's all shift – they definitely weren't flattering. Thus, the

 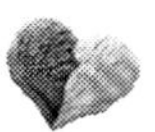

slightest imperfect area of one's body – big boobs, big tummy, big thighs – all looked bigger in scrubs.

I was the head nurse of the unit at the time, known and respected by all the medical staff. And I knew and respected all of them. When one day I was in close proximity to Dr. Smith, one of the older docs who'd worked there forever. He was checking on his babies who were to be discharged.

"So when's the baby due?" he asked me as he was examining one of his bundles of joy who was due to go home that day.

"Pardon me?" I queried, holding my breath, certain he hadn't just asked me what I thought he'd asked me. Because ooops – guess what? I wasn't pregnant!

He took the stethoscope out of his ears, pulled the baby's undershirt back down, and tucked the little cutie back in his blanket. He smiled at me, as if already congratulating me, while my stomach and Miss Mojo were doing the flop-de-flop.

Now what you've got to know about Dr. Smith is that he was probably 70 years old, had practiced at that same hospital for 40 years, was always super nice to everybody – especially the staff. He even dressed up as Santa for Christmas every year since he had the belly and the bushy eyebrows to wear the costume. Bottom line? Everybody loved him. He would never intentionally hurt anyone. And little did he know he'd just sliced and diced Miss Mojo to pieces.

So when he asked me that, I wanted to cold cock him then and there, but he was just too much of a sweetheart to pounce back at with nails bared. I swallowed my pride, gulped down the extra saliva that had built up in my mouth, and attempted a smile, which I'm sure came out like a crooked smirk instead, and calmly replied, "Nope, Dr. Smith. No baby cooking here."

I stared at him, hoping I was giving him yet another version of "the look." As in, "I surely hope you understand just how hurtful your well meant words were. I can't believe after this many years you still haven't learned how not to stick your foot in your mouth, asking women anything about a pregnancy of any kind!"

He replied, "Well, what's wrong with having a bun in the oven?" He moved on to his next baby on his list of discharges. "Making a baby is the most wonderful gift from God," he added. He glanced up at the ceiling then, as if having a little conversation with God above, right that second. "Just look around at all these little miracles," he said, waving to all the babies in the unit.

He put his stethoscope back into his ears to listen to the next child, a little girl, all dressed in pink, who started to cry emphatically when the cold stethoscope met the warmth of her skin. He talked to her gently and made goo-goo sounds to help quiet her down, rocking her body gently with his free hand.

While I would have loved to get into a royal bitch session with him, for sexual harassment or pure stupidity when it comes to what things one simply doesn't ever say to a woman, it just wouldn't have been right. He was a sweetheart with one of the biggest hearts in any man you'd ever meet. I wasn't going to change him.

He was right about just how miraculous life really is. He went back to talking baby talk to his little one, rocking her again with his free hand, and I went back to what I had been working on before he'd arrived and asked me that question.

Miss Mojo hated us that day. But it wasn't long before that would change. Dr. Smith's words had gotten to me – to at least

 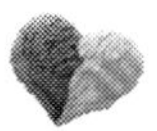

get back in a fitness mindset. Right after that, I signed up for an aerobics class and loved it – back in the days of Jane Fonda and "feel the burn." I ended up eventually teaching the class, which really kept me on track with my own weight and fitness for quite some time to come.

While I wasn't with child when Dr. Smith made that comment, I did get pregnant a bit farther down the road. It came at a time when I was busy with my life as a nurse and part-time aerobics instructor and Kevin was moving up in the banking world.

Ironically, this was one of the rare times in my life that I did not have to worry about my weight. But my obstetrician was after me about it constantly. Not for the reasons you might think. He wasn't giving me the lecture that eating for two was not an excuse to eat everything in my path and gain 50 pounds, which is what most of my friends were struggling with. His lecture to me was that I needed to gain more! I have to admit that struck a nerve, recalling my 7-Eleven debacle.

My first trimester had been a nightmare, full of nausea and vomiting, and the second wasn't much better. I could barely keep any food down. It didn't help that I was working the night shift at the time, which screwed up morning sickness for me even more, as my body must have thought that mornings for me were when I would wake at around four or five p.m. after sleeping all day. Even the sight or smell of food made me throw up. Kevin and I couldn't even eat together for several of those months. And the smell of pizza? I simply had to leave the house.

I got pregnant weighing 150 pounds and I instantly lost 7 tossing my cookies all the time. The only time I could eat was when I got off work at 7 a.m., when I was ravenous and would eat like I was eating for a dozen babies.

The cook at the hospital made these amazing huge blueberry pancakes, smothered in butter and slathered with syrup, which I savored each morning. On top of that I'd devour some bacon, hash browns, and a large orange juice, probably consuming close to 3,000 calories each morning. But the rest of the day I just couldn't eat without it coming back up. At one point my doc suggested I eat peanut butter because it was hard for it to come back up! I admit it did help a bit.

Then, the worst night of all, about four months into the pregnancy, when the nausea and vomiting seemed to be gone and I actually had a craving for fast food – I got food poisoning. I didn't know which end to put where as both my stomach and my intestines were not happy for quite some time. I nearly went to the hospital, probably should have, but things finally settled down and I made it through the night. Over the weeks I gradually started putting some of my weight back on. By the time I weighed in at the doc's office the day before I delivered I weighed 163#. Only 13 pounds from my starting weight. But the first day after I delivered I was back to my pre-pregnancy weight of 150#. It was a hell of a way to lose weight!

And so we became parents of a beautiful baby daughter. She came with a full head of black hair (which would fade to blonde), brilliant blue eyes just like her dad, and all the right parts in the right places. She also was a very easy baby. We thought she was perfect. She even fit well into our active lifestyle, going hiking with us tucked into a Snugli or, as soon as she was old enough, taking bike rides with us in her baby

 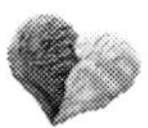

bike seat. She also slept through the night when she was only a few weeks old. We were very spoiled!

We named her Shaun. It was the only name we could agree upon, be it boy or girl. (Back in 1983 they still didn't know what the sex was until a baby actually came into the world.) Considering it's still predominately a man's world, and likely still will be for years to come, her name has served her well as a doctor and surgeon, especially when folks are choosing their doctors based on their names in the Yellow Pages. Even today in her practice she has patients say, "I was expecting a man," when she shows up and introduces herself as their surgeon. She bites her tongue and tries to smile, but it's kind of like the pregnancy question. Just not appropriate.

On top of juggling our busy careers and a new baby, I also attended graduate school part time for two years and got my master's degree in pediatric nursing. Can you spell "over-achiever"?

It's truly amazing what you can fit into a busy life when you have to!

* * *

I always figured when I went to nursing school that I would be a bedside nurse all my life, but as they say, "Life is what happens when you make other plans," and that sure applied to us.

After 7-1/2 years of nursing and acquiring my master's degree, an opportunity opened up that I never expected ... I became a medical sales rep for Imed Corporation, one of the major manufacturers of IV pumps in the country. I was the only rep for them in the Colorado and Wyoming territory, worked out of my home office, and was occasionally on the road for several days at a time. I remember feeling like my heart was torn out of me when I was required to attend training in San Diego for two weeks. I'd never been away from Shaun for that long and although she was only four years old, she learned pretty quickly that two weeks was a very long time. She still remembers that time today.

It was quite a change for me, being one of a half dozen females in the sales force. I'd gone from working with 99 percent women, to something like 90 percent men. And most of them very competitive, very handsome, (and they knew it) and narcissistic as well. While Miss Mojo was learning to handle most situations, in that world I didn't even know what I didn't know about workplace mis-behaviors. Sexual harassment was in its early days of just being recognized, much less being dealt with. No one even knew there was such a thing as emotional abuse yet.

I remember one time when I was still very new to the job and was on the phone with the top dog of the company. He was griping at me about some account or other and how everything must have been my fault that things weren't going well there. He was literally shouting at me over the phone. I was already a heap on the floor, feeling horrible, sitting there taking his mental whipping, when all at once he stopped and the phone line went dead. I let out a huge sigh of relief, certain that he must have gotten cut off somehow, when I realized that he had just put me on speaker phone for all the folks in his office to hear. Then, he started blasting me again for my inept behavior! He was indeed a master in the art of emotional

 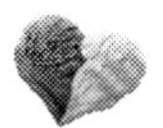

abuse. The part he didn't understand is that I have always done better with a carrot than a stick, when I'm needing encouragement or have done something wrong. Emotional beating and embarrassments do NOT make me perform better.

To make things worse, these early days of sexual harassment still went mostly unreported, as I quickly learned.

The clothes didn't help – I wore suits and dresses and tailored skirts and blouses ... a far cry from baggy scrubs – the ones Dr. Smith said I looked pregnant in. About that time my body was in pretty great shape as well ... despite having had a baby. And I seemed to attract the attention of a rather handsome gentleman named Jack Johnson.

I remember a rather uncomfortable evening sitting next to him at an awards banquet held to honor the highest hitters in the sales force. He was perhaps in his mid-50's, only about 5'7" or so, but very fit and with a full head of absolutely gorgeous white hair, with a beautifully styled salt and pepper goatee. He reminded me of Jay Leno, both with the interesting hair-do and the fact that he had Jay's personality. He was the class clown, the life of the party, and the king of sexual harassment, unbeknownst to me. But I sure as hell knew by the end of the night.

Later, he ended up sitting behind me and would occasionally lean forward to whisper something in my ear. It started as just telling me some personal tidbit about one of the winners. "He's got twin boys at home that are star athletes." I thought that was nice. Then he moved on to commenting on the (few) female reps who were being called up. "God, she's in great shape, isn't she?" came his next commentary. He'd been drinking heavily all evening and his inhibitions were disappearing minute by minute.

Then a gal named Claudia went up to receive her plaque and his eyes couldn't stop following her as she floated in a stunning, very form-fitting, floor-length black gown. She was smiling and shaking the big boss's hand as the audience clapped when he whispered in my ear, "She's gained some weight this year and it all went to her butt. I absolutely love that woman's bootie, don't you?"

I could feel myself freeze up, not knowing what to do with that. He recognized my discomfort – hell, he'd created it – and he went on to see just how far he could go before he got a rise out of me. "I bet your bootie's better than that," he whispered, then patted my shoulders gently, as if we'd been intimate already. "You've obviously got better boobs than she does." (There it was again – that ridiculous belief of so many men, believing we women order our boobs out of a catalogue. And that we well-endowed gals ordered our boobs in size large so that we could attract boob men with them.

I felt like yelling at him, "No, you asshole, that's just where my extra fat goes when I gain more weight than I need."

Instead, I felt myself stiffen and the hair on the back of my neck stand up. Here I was at a big company gig, with a guy who held a very high position, who was coming on to me. And me – still not very worldly – trying to figure out my options and to try not to make a scene.

The last thing he said before I got up and left the room was, "I bet you're getting wet down there, aren't you? But I'm not sure if that's for me or for her?"

I grabbed my purse and excused myself to my table mates and went to my room without explanation.

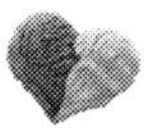

That next morning my boss knocked on my door, to check in on me. His name was Jim and he was the best boss you could ever ask for. Funny, kind, compassionate. He'd seen me leave the night before and thought I hadn't felt well. When I explained the situation to him, I could see his expression change to a face filled with anger. "I'm so sorry, MJ. I'll talk to Jack about his behavior. I promise you, he'll never bother you again."

The long and the short of it was that Jack was told to leave me alone. Period. No reprimand. Not even a slap on the wrist. Certainly no apology. Nothing that might teach him that his behavior could get him (and the company) in trouble in the future.

Fortunately, he wasn't someone who I would be around often, so I didn't have to worry much on that score. However, on the rare times that I did see him, he'd always smile, then wink at me, enough to say, "Nobody can hurt me, Baby. I'm invincible." And I suspect he was right. All I know is that he was still in his high-powered job for years after I left. Wonder how many other women he harassed? I suspect few ever reported him, sad as that is ...

* * *

What a fine line we walk with weight. Weigh too much and you're fat and easily made fun of. Weigh just right and you're sexy and "asking for it," in terms of sexual attractiveness. Weigh too little and people think you're sick or that you look like a boy or perhaps you're gay. Is it any wonder so many women are confused as to what a healthy weight is? And with situations like the one just mentioned, is it any wonder that some women gain weight just so jerks like him will leave them alone?

It was a pretty stressful job, even without having to worry about idiots like Jack. In fact, we had 60 sales reps to cover the whole country and 30% of them quit every year. I lasted nearly eight years. While it was nice having my office at home and my boss several states away, the job, with its travel requirements, was pretty hard on the family life.

However, it was also pretty lucrative if you were good at it and had the perseverance to put in the time and the work. I did and I did. I even slept in a hospital bed several nights, making sure that the nurses, no matter what shift they worked, knew how to use my machines.

In the long run, I won a huge account which, combined with my husband's job – by then a VP of a large investment firm – ironically I was able to put my fancy suits in the back of the closet and pull out my jeans! Finally, we bought a small ranch on five acres about 20 miles outside of Denver and got into horses big time! I'd never forgotten my time with Queenie and could finally buy horses of my own and couldn't wait to teach Shaun how to ride.

The dreams of a horsie kid were fast coming true.

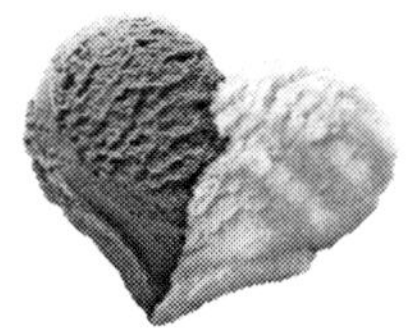

CHAPTER 6

Horsing Around

The next several years, living on a ranch, were the best years of my life.

I had little trouble with my weight back then, despite the fact that I was still a closet sugar junkie and I still weighed myself every day. I certainly didn't teach my daughter healthy eating concepts either. She's reminded me of at least one occasion (likely many more) when I served her leftover birthday cake for breakfast! But, fortunately, the daily chores and endless hours in the saddle were now our workouts. Plus, you carry around enough 60-pound bales of hay day after day and shovel horse manure that never ends and you build some pretty strong biceps too.

Our home in Parker, Colorado was all we'd ever dreamed of. It had a large, two-story house, a small, four-stall barn, and five acres where the horses got to graze a good deal of the time. There were only 40 houses in the entire subdivision with everyone owning approximately five acres per plot. About 40 percent of them had horses. The others just loved the open space and the privacy that allowed.

The land was a high plain, desert-like, with sharp-edged yucca plants everywhere and a handful of ponderosa pine trees scattered across the properties. The wind had little to stop it, which meant in the summer we almost always had a nice breeze, and in the winter we were certain to have huge drifts we'd always need to dig out from. There was a small outdoor riding arena and several jumps set up in the pasture where we would practice jumping, many of them made with barrels, piles of wood, and even tires.

Sprawling through the middle of the community was a huge sand gully that 98 percent of the year was bone dry sand. However, the other 2 percent, after a huge rain, was a flash flood zone, where all the water from neighboring properties drained into it, turning it into a surging, dangerous river, big enough and powerful enough to carry a semi-truck with it. As such, it was in a flood zone so no one could build on it.

But we could ride on it, whenever we wanted. It was acres and acres of open fields, with a long, sloping hill that was awesome to gallop up. There were occasionally a few pronghorn antelope who would pass through the area. And a small herd of deer lived there, pretty much year round.

Did I mention that Kevin was allergic to horses? While he had learned to ride when he was a kid, his allergies to horses and hay didn't kick in until he got older and at our new home he stayed away from the barn as much as possible, although he would ride with us on occasion, loading up on allergy pills beforehand. More often, he'd head to the golf course and we'd all share stories of our day's activities over the dinner table.

Shaun and I lived and breathed horses – in fact I built a small business, buying and selling horses. I would usually buy them off the race track when their age sent them to retirement from the racing world, and we would teach them to jump,

 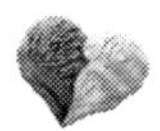

then find a new home for them in the horse show world. If I was lucky I might net a few bucks but not much.

It was a labor of love and one I was thrilled to share with my daughter. She was riding by age 7 and stayed with it until she went out of state to medical school at age 22. I still laugh remembering her first horse show. We went with a friend to a small, backyard show that was about as low-key as you can get. Shaun was the only kid who was under age ten signed up to compete in the only class for youngsters. Normally, the class would be cancelled without six competitors or so, but the judge decided to let her enter anyway since it was the only class she was old enough to enter. Nervous as hell but having figured out the situation just as she was about to enter the arena, she turned to me and asked, "I'm going to win a blue ribbon no matter what I do, aren't I?"

One smart kid. I smiled back and said, "Just have fun," as she nudged the horse with her heels and made a little clicking sound with her tongue, and the little chestnut-colored mare named Sundown headed out to the center of the ring. The judge directed Shaun to walk and trot in both directions and in the end, handed her a blue ribbon. (One of so many she would win over the years.)

That day, she knew she'd win no matter what, but the joy of putting herself out there in that empty arena, at age 7 one-on-one with that judge, was something that not every kid could do. And she pulled it off with confidence. Talk about one of those little Miss Mojo moments.

By the time she was ten she had won, on her own merits, a regional championship in jumping, and continued to compete in jumping and dressage events for years. I'd taken on the competitive circuit myself and sometimes Shaun and I even competed against each other and, believe me, I didn't always win.

My own riding improved as well. I'd gone from being a purely Western rider who had spent all those years leading dudes around, to a jumper, and I loved the power I felt steering my 1,400-pound horse, Murphy, over a big, solid jump nearly four feet high. We were a team. My job was to point him to which jump came next and his job was to get us over it. Miss Mojo was overjoyed each time I edged up my degree of difficulty and was successful in doing so. I have to admit not all of those experiences were positive. I'd definitely hit the ground numerous times. (As had Shaun. It simply comes with the territory.) The hardest part was getting back on – especially if I'd been hurt. But the confidence we both built over time was a priceless gift for facing many tough situations that would face us ahead in life.

In addition to competing as an individual, Shaun joined a local chapter of the United States Pony Club, an international equestrian organization where most of our Olympic equestrians got their basics. They didn't just teach riding, they taught knowledge pertaining to horse care, along with teamwork, responsibility, stick-to-it-ive-ness, and so much more. Whenever they competed they did so as a team, with one person as a stable manager, responsible for keeping everyone organized, on time, and making sure the horses and all their tack and equipment were properly cared for as well. Parents were strictly forbidden to go into the barns while the kids learned how to do things for themselves, with minimal supervision from the barn judges.

 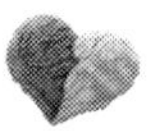

Boy, did those kids learn priceless life lessons. While anyone can be supportive when experiencing the thrill of victory, when the agony of defeat happens, it takes a team to sometimes pull someone who'd had a bad day back out of the sadness. Horses don't always do what we expect they'll do and the rider can suffer the consequences. Falling off, getting eliminated for making a mistake, or having your horse refuse a jump over and over can all ruin your day. But these kids not only helped each other, they were becoming good, strong team players at the same time.

Recently while in the midst of moving, I was going through some boxes of stuff from our horsie days and found a letter that a mom had written to Shaun years ago thanking her for taking her daughter under her wing and giving her a compassionate pep talk after she'd been eliminated for one reason or another. The mother explained just how much Shaun's compassion had meant to the much younger girl, who thought she'd just been dealt the worst day of her life. The experience was priceless, to both girls, I think. One of those life lessons that you just can't create if you tried.

Our times together were priceless. I think our favorite times were the ones when we just rode together on the sandy trails of the flood plane behind our property. I especially recall cantering up the big hill that made the horses work a little but kept the gallop one that was not too fast or too slow. It took several minutes to get to the top of the small hill, and all four of us were usually winded and breathing hard once we got there. Then, as we'd all catch our breath a bit, we'd always admire the vista from there.

With no buildings or trees to obliterate the view, we could see 20 miles or more in each direction, with a spectacular view of the entire mountain range, usually still covered with snow. Looking north we could barely make out the sky scrapers of downtown Denver. Mostly we admired the wide-open spaces on all sides that we were blessed with. I think even the horses loved that particular exercise, as they always fought to see who would reach the top first. It was like having our own little piece of heaven.

We also spent hundreds of hours in the barn grooming and feeding and picking up after the horses, as well as hauling them in the trailer to compete or participate in clinics. Those long hours working or on the trails were some of the best times we've ever spent. We even slept in our horse trailer together when an event was far from home, and it was a small enough space that you had to snuggle up or you just wouldn't fit. What mom doesn't value every snuggle minute she can get, even when her kids aren't little any more?

* * *

Of course not everything in life is happy. Sometimes things come in goods and bads. And when the bads came, my personal therapy came in the forms of sugar, chocolate, ice cream, and all the rest. Which doesn't fix the problem; just puts a band aid on it. Some problems just have no answer – only pain. And only time will heal them.

And when the bad thing hits your kid, it's even worse. In April of 1996, it hit us hard …

Shaun was 13 at the time. Just old enough to start thinking she was all grown up but clueless just how far from grown up she was! Age 13 was when her pretty, happy little life got

 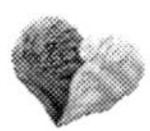

turned upside down, as did all of ours. But when you're the parents, you've got to the be strong ones for your kids. And that's no easy job either.

It started out with a sudden and unexpected death in the family, which stopped all of us in our tracks. Shaun's aunt, Michele, only in her mid-40's, died, leaving us all lacking for words to explain such confusing concepts to Shaun and her two young cousins. Answering the "whys." Reassuring the young ones that they were safe and loved and wouldn't die themselves any minute. Trying to understand the unfamiliar looks on the grownups faces. The kids were confused, lost, and terrified.

Michele had died on a Saturday and the funeral was planned for the following Wednesday. We all tried to bear up over the next several days. We were going through the motions of life as usual when Monday morning I heard screaming from Shaun's room. I flew out of bed, with Kevin right behind me, for the sound of that kind of screaming had to mean something awful. I figured it was a nightmare, but it was so much worse.

She was crying and screaming, "Banana's dead! Banana's dead!" Sobbing her eyes out as she held up her little hamster she'd named Bananas, lifeless in her hands. Kevin and I looked at each other with wordless expressions that said, "Really, God? You really had to do this right now?" My eyes filled up with tears as well, as I wracked my brain with how we should handle this new crisis when we hadn't finished the first one yet.

Needless to say it was a tough morning with so many tears and even more questions about God and heaven and death.

The house seemed hauntingly quiet as no one knew what to say and even the mandatory phone calls to make all the funeral arrangements seemed to be done in whispers.

Shaun found a beautiful little gift box to place Bananas in and we took him out to the far corner of the pasture which, over time, ended up becoming the pet cemetery for a few other small creatures who spent their short lives with us as well. She put some flowers on his grave and we all cried again, then had to start preparing ourselves for Michele's funeral on Wednesday.

It was a Catholic, open-casket ceremony and I could see that the kids were so confused about the whole concept of death. Hell, so were the adults. But the kids – they were simply lost. And staring at their aunt's body in the coffin was just beyond their comprehension. All we could do was be there for them. Thank God we made it through that day. By the time Wednesday was over, we all just wanted to get back to our routines with the hope of finding something comforting within them.

So when Thursday rolled around, Shaun headed back to school and she and Kevin were scheduled to see an Avalanche hockey game that night. I didn't expect them to get home until 10:30 or so. I hoped that hockey would at least take their minds off of all the stress of the week for a little while.

As for me – it was time to take a nice, long trail ride and see if I couldn't find a quiet place at the top of our galloping hill to feel closer to God.

So I headed to the barn and decided to ride our newest horse, which Shaun had named Calvin Kline. We'd only found him a couple of months before but we were very excited about him already. He was copper-penny red with four beautiful

 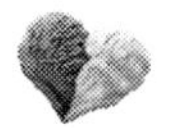

white, matching stockings to the knee and a big, white blaze down his face. On his left hip he displayed an unusual brand with some unspecified code.

He wasn't very tall but his body was the perfect size for Shaun, who wasn't very tall herself. He had a very gentle demeanor, seemed very easy going, and was pretty darned broke. But what made him so special was that this horse didn't just trot – he floated. No, more accurately – he danced. He literally moved as if he were a ballet dancer, with each trot step suspending him in the air for just a little bit longer than most any horse around. In the world of dressage riding (think dancing horses competing in dancing competitions) he was a natural – but also a diamond in the rough.

I'd bought him through an auction for next to nothing and had tracked down his brand through the Colorado Brand Office, and through that, to a previous owner who said he'd been a cow pony and had only chased cows for a living. The cowboy didn't even know what the heck *dressage* was. And Calvin, we would soon discover, didn't even know what grain was. But he sure learned right quick.

It didn't take much to get him ready for his first little show, just to see how he'd handle the hubbub and all that goes with horse-showing. He did just fine. And in fact, Shaun came in 3rd place with him, which was way outside our realm of what we'd thought was possible, all things considered. We even got a couple of great photos of him dancing with Shaun, which was awesome evidence of his abilities. The show season ahead was going to be very exciting.

So, that day, for my morning ride to hopefully find some solace in the great outdoors, I chose Calvin. It was beautiful spring weather. None of the horses had been ridden over the last few difficult days and he seemed quite happy meandering along the trail at his usual slow-poke pace. I waved at my neighbor Mike, a retired military guy, who was fussing in his garden as usual, but there was no one else to be seen for as far as the eye could see on that Thursday morning. Most people were at work by then and wouldn't be home for hours. And Kevin and Shaun weren't due in until late that evening. The day was mine.

We wandered through the sand gully for quite a while, watching a hawk soar above us as he searched for a lunch of rabbit or snake or prairie dog. The sky was filled with diminishing, white jet contrails from planes that had recently flown over us. Those white contrails always looked to me like a child had been painting stripes in the sky.

The peacefulness I always felt out on this rugged, natural terrain was such a blessing. There were tiny flowers everywhere as it was spring. Blue ones, red ones, yucca's with their white seed pods waiting to burst open. The shape and curves of the gully itself changed after every substantial rain that came along. On one side of me it was perhaps 15 feet high and the sand was of various colors, leaving patterns in the wall itself. Then it leveled out, turning into that deep, deep kind of sand on an empty beach somewhere. The kind you worked your butt off on trying to walk through. Then, on the far side of the beach sand area, the land gradually ascended again, into a long ridge that climbed for a couple of miles or so.

That was where the galloping hill was and I aimed Calvin right for it, knowing it would be the best part of the outing. I nudged him with my heels and kissed to him to wake him up and he picked up the pace to his slow, steady canter. He didn't

 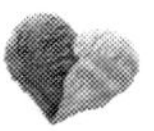

have a speedy bone in his body, so I was prepared for his usual twiddle-your-thumbs kind of pace.

He was so much fun to ride, with that smooth, dancing gait. I felt as if I was one with him at that moment. I leaned slightly forward in the saddle to make it easier for him to carry me, and heard his rhythmical breathing, "Whoosh, whoosh," as he took each stride. I could feel his powerful muscles straining as he ascended the moderate grade and as he dug down deep for the power to make it to the top.

All at once I felt a huge jolt. A "thump" of sorts, and I felt my body start leaning suddenly towards the left. My brain was instantly trying to figure out what was going on and all I could think of was that he'd perhaps stepped in some kind of hole and broken his leg.

It all seemed like it happened in slow motion and as if it all was taking place on a big screen in some movie theatre with me watching the show and waiting for the save-the-day ending that always happens in the very last seconds of all those feel-good movies.

Only it was real. I kept hold of the reins in my right hand and flew off of Calvin from his left side, just in time to see him stagger to the right and collapse in a heap in front of me, his breath pouring out of him in one giant rush as his thousand-pound body went slamming onto the ground beneath. As I gasped to catch my breath and tried to figure out what the hell happened, he let out one small nicker and a drop of blood fell from his nostril. Then nothing. His body lay motionless. That beautiful red coat, those flashy white stockings and blaze, and those incredible dancing legs – perfectly still.

I must have been in shock. My brain couldn't take it all in. I just stood there, unable to move. Gasping for breath. The adrenaline pumping through me so fiercely that I was shaking from head to toe as hot tears started coming like rain. And all I remember saying, shouting, was "No, no, no ... you can't do this to her too."

I paced around for a few minutes, keeping a watch on his nostrils; praying with all my might that any second he'd start breathing again. "Come on, Calvin," I yelled at him, "Please, please, please don't go." I screamed at the top of my lungs then, realizing that no one could possible hear me. Not even Mike, who by this time was a few miles away.

I kneeled down next to him then and stroked his neck and his face and spoke to him gently. Then realizing the outbursts had taken all of me that I had to spare … and I still had to get back home. All the while the tears kept rushing. My thoughts still: What was I going to tell Shaun?

Then I realized something else. Had I not jumped off of him when I did, I could have died too. Or even worse, I could have lain there for hours stuck underneath him with no one having a clue where I was until possibly the next day… or later. That vision stuck with me for quite some time.

I cried all the way back home and was grateful to still find Mike out in the garden where I blubbered the story to him. He gave me his shoulder to cry on, then got me back home where he called my trainer who came right away. Then I called Kevin. His secretary told me he was at the company's attorney's office and when I told her it was an emergency, she tracked him down for me. When he came on the phone I was blubbering again and between my sobs he could barely make out me saying that someone else had died.

"Who died now?" I could sense the fear in his voice.

 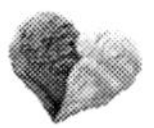

I tried to slow my breathing down enough to tell him it was Calvin, then went back to uncontrollable sobbing. The whole ordeal still too raw and just too unbelievable.

I knew he was as fried as I was after the week we'd had and now the realization that we had a kid at home who'd already been given enough for one week, and had just been handed this, as well. Kevin too was lost. We agreed that he'd still take her to the hockey game and at least get one relaxing evening before we had to share this news with her.

What Calvin died of that day wasn't ever one hundred percent clear. He was a young horse. About equivalent to a twenty-something year old person. The best the vet could guess was that he'd blown an aneurism. Whatever it was, I hope when it's my time to go it is just that quick without pain or suffering. Although it sure is tough on those left behind.

As you might guess, things were pretty horrific for a while for us. Time is the only ointment that can help heal a wound that deep. Although food doesn't hurt. But neither time nor food was enough for quite some time. I dove into baking. Cookies being my usual favorites. Chocolate chip, of course. Rice Krispies treats were always a stand-by. Candy bars were a daily fix. Things settled down over time but not without a new level of weight around my middle. I don't think I even weighed myself then. I just didn't care.

* * *

And life went on, as it always does. Although it took both Shaun and me some time to find our Mojo again. Confidence takes so long to build and can be so quickly shattered. But with new horses who came along and new competitions and horse shows to partake in, we'd gotten back in our usual routines. Murphy and I had even been making some real strides in our jumping abilities, which was never easy with him because it was often an argument as to who was in charge. It was such a fine line I walked with him. But, bit by bit, we had been making headway and were jumping some four-foot fences that were pretty daunting but pretty breathtaking when we mastered them.

My trainer, Gwen, had encouraged me to enter the Appaloosa World Show in Dallas in October. She really thought we were ready and that I could kick some serious butt. And, as it was only August, I should have plenty of time to put on the finishing touches to get ready.

Yet, just when I started giving it serious thought, life had other plans again. My father, who had suffered from Alzheimer's for many years, had fallen into a coma and wasn't expected to last long. I flew back home to Wisconsin immediately, where I did vigil with my mother for nearly a week, before my father left this life for the next one.

That week was exhausting. Anyone who has sat with someone in a coma who is preparing to pass knows exactly what I mean. The life he'd been in for so many years, lost in his own dark and cloudy thoughts and images, was certainly not the way that he had ever envisioned his last days on this planet. Nor for us either.

My mother and I grew closer over those days. How could we not after experiencing what we shared together? We were both there with him until he passed. All the rest of my family came in for the viewing and the funeral and there was a large

 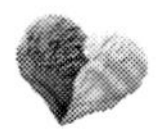

number of people from Whitewater who had known my dad for years, who showed up to pay their respects as well.

By the time I flew home I was consumed with depression and ate everything in my path – at least when I wasn't sleeping, which was my other escape from the pain. I even remember one day in particular taking a tablespoon to a bag of brown sugar and just eating it straight. You'd think at least I could have had a sugar rush, but no such luck. I was just numb.

The only happiness I found was on the back of my horse. But most of the time I simply couldn't stir up enough energy to even do that.

Murphy seemed to know that he needed to be gentle with me for a awhile. We did some quiet trail riding now and then, when I could get myself out of bed long enough to ride. Finally, my trainer felt she had given me enough time to grieve and gave me a swift kick in the butt to get me back in gear.

"There's still a few days before entries are due for the World Show in Dallas, MJ. If you put your mind to it and you two start pushing yourselves a bit, you've got all the reasons in the world to win this thing."

I argued with her up one side and down the other, but in the end she must have reached my reclusive Miss Mojo and convinced her that this was our year – and, believe it or not, it was! I finally took the big step, for my next adventure, and sent in my entry. So we both worked our butts off, practicing every combination of complicated jumps that Gwen could think of. Finally, I loaded Murphy in the trailer and we headed down the road. He handled the long trip to Dallas as if it was just a few blocks from home. And he performed like a star in the ring, jumping any jump I pointed him at (without argument), and I let him be in charge once I pointed out his next fence for him. The competition was tough and the fences were complicated with some tight corners, all of which he sailed over. We were an unstoppable team!

I felt like I was flying again. That we were truly a team. That nothing was impossible. That my Mojo had indeed come out of hiding after so long away. At that moment I knew that I could do anything, even after all that I'd been through.

We headed home champions and brought home some incredible bronze trophies to prove it.

It was a good thing that Miss Mojo had returned, because besides all the usual reasons, it ended up that I was going to need all she could give me and then some over the next few years.

But for that amazing week far away from home, I started to realize that it's my adventurous spirit that must always be fed, or else my addictive side will always win out.

CHAPTER 7

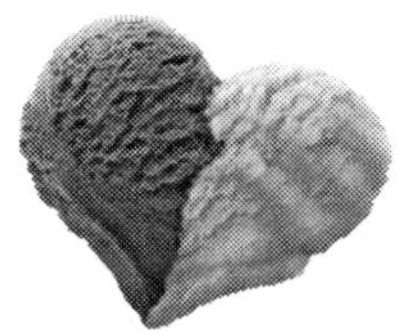

Running Away From Home—As An Adult

"Till death do us part," we had promised each other on June 24, 1978. But people change over time. Relationships change. And boy, do marriages change. After 25 years together, we left our lives as we had known them, and went through the dark days of divorce. We'd waited until Shaun had headed off to college, but the pain and circumstances that still took place impacted everything we did. Including four years of counseling. Essentially we called it "irreconcilable differences."

However, walking away from a 25-year relationship was not done lightly nor without guilt or second thoughts.

That doesn't mean that the process was easy. In fact, it was the worst time in my life, and likely was for Kevin as well.

Emotions were high and sensitivities even higher. The smallest slight felt like the deepest wound. Boundaries were drawn in the sand. Arguments about who got what were painful. And all of this happened on the heels of the disaster at the World Trade Center, which left our entire nation in a world of fear, sadness, anger, pain, and depression. My own depression had moved in over the last couple of years, with no plans of moving out anytime soon, while I was struggling with the unravelling of the marriage. Add the dark, freezing days of winter settling in and I was an emotional wreck. In fact, I was suicidal.

I just couldn't see an end to the pain. And for anyone who has ever wondered how someone could take their own life, know this: they simply want the pain to stop and are in such a dark place that they cannot see alternative ways of making that happen.

My friends knew I was a mess; they just didn't realize how bad I was. (I had actually written my suicide letter already ... they had no idea.) And they gently suggested I take a vacation somewhere. Get away from it all. Get some well-deserved rest in some place far away from the emotional war zone I was living in.

"How would you like to go somewhere?" my friend and boss, Deb, probed, while we were at lunch one gloomy November day. I was eating the most enormous piece of molten lava cake that was designed to be shared but which I kept close so that no one else would get any of my addictive drug. At least sugar still gave me an occasional but temporary rush.

I shrugged my shoulders, apathetic.

Now my friend Lynn joined in: "Have you got your own credit card?"

They looked at each other, then back to me, then back to each other. I could tell they had some plan a brewin'.

I nodded again, wondering where this was going.

"Have you got any room on it?" Deb went on.

 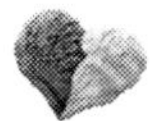

Once again, a subtle nod from me, and perhaps a tiny skip of my heart as I was starting to get the plan they had thought up for me.

"It's dirt cheap to fly right now," Deb reminded me. "You could get away for a week for peanuts."

"And we'll even take care of the horses for you," Lynn added. They let me think about it but only for a moment. Then Lynn came back with ... "So, where would you like to go?"

"Somewhere warm where I could dive," I heard myself whisper. And Cozumel, Mexico came to mind.

And so, on Thanksgiving Day 2001, I found myself on a plane to Cozumel. A very empty plane, I might add, as people were still worried about terrorism and were traveling as little as possible. Even the hotel occupancy rate was hovering around 30 percent, which was OK with me. I wasn't ready for a bunch of wild, screaming kids. I was hoping for some sun, a lot of sleeping on the beach, the sound of some waves, and maybe a SCUBA dive, if I felt up to it. I had brought my gear along, being optimistic.

However, I wasn't too excited about displaying my body in a bathing suit right then. I was hanging around 175 pounds and hadn't really cared what I'd put in my mouth for some time.

But then I thought, "Who gives a crap?" and pulled out my old stand-by one-piece tank suit that accommodated me at quite a wide range of weights. It would have to do.

I had been to Cozumel once, years before when Shaun was 12 and we'd gone there as a family to get certified in SCUBA diving. Cozumel is a small island, about 28 miles long and 12 miles wide; a 30-minute ferry ride from Playa del Carmen on the mainland. Cancun is just 45 minutes due north from there.

The island touts only one small town, San Miguel, where the boat docks attract both ferries, which depart hourly, moving locals and tourists alike from the island to the mainland, and the enormous cruise ships that dump their hoards of shoppers, bicyclists, and *turistas* to participate in a wide variety of activities on the island six days a week. It is a hustling little town every day but Sundays, when no cruise ships stop. On its regular business days the little town is full of color, energy, and as many Let's-Make-A-Deal slick Mexican salesmen as each street could hold. Tourists are easy targets as they unload from the ferry or ship that brought them to the island. The local sales guys look at each new boat bringing "fresh meat" – unsuspecting folks who had just come for a day of wandering around the town, yet somehow always end up with toys, treasures, and tours they hadn't planned on.

Once a would-be victim gets past the activity hawkers (snorkeling, diving, jeep jungle tours), the next layer of pitchers are the folks who ran the diamond and other high-end merchandise stores. Each standing outside their shop, directing all who come their way into their cool, air conditioned place filled with baubles every tourist simply has to go home with.

And if you could get past those wheeler-dealers, the last layer of shop-keepers are those who hock the lower end merchandise – from all sorts of silver jewelry, to Oakley sunglasses impostors, to huge bottles of vanilla, to t-shirts, to the always in-demand items like prescription drugs (available

 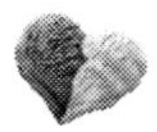

there without prescriptions), to the all-time-standby, Tequila – duty free!

Sunday nights all the local people come out to the town plaza to celebrate with their families and friends, share food and drink and music. A local band playing all the Latin favorites keeps the rhythm and the energy up as dancers, young and old, turn out in their most colorful dress-up clothes. Some of the women wear the traditional long dresses with the lace edging and bold, rainbow colors. Others are clad in the traditional pure-white dress with a colorful sash, yet never a spot of dirt on them.

Grand babies dance with grandpas. Senior couples who had been together for decades and knew each other so well that they danced if they were one, dance one dance after the next after the next – defying all odds of being tired at their age. Three and four-year-olds running in and out between the dancers, screaming and giggling, all adding up to a cultural energy that keeps them all dancing, eating, and drinking (mostly alcohol) into the wee hours.

But that was the Cozumel I remembered from our family trip. This time, no cruise ships docked in the harbor. Few people got off the ferry for a day of exploring the island. Many shops appeared to be closed for good. Most of the workers had no idea how they would feed their families during this world-wide panic due to September 11th. I noticed the change as soon as the taxi picked me up at the airport and drove me through the downtown area on the way to my hotel.

I felt almost ashamed that I was bitching and moaning about my circumstances at home when these people had nothing and no idea when things might change. Moreover, I felt horrible that I had been so close to taking my own life for reasons that felt totally justified at the moment, but now seemed so miniscule.

Spending that week in paradise turned out to be the best decision of my life. The weight called stress that I carried like an anvil around my neck, immediately lifted upon arriving in that wonderful, tropical paradise with its sunshine, surf, and sea. I suddenly felt like I was being swaddled in a warm blanket on a freezing, cold night. I had never vacationed by myself before. Travel on business alone, sure. Vacation? Nope. It felt weird. But with each passing day I began to feel like I might actually be able to turn my depression around and find a contentedness again.

I put a lot into those seven days. I spent hours just sleeping on a lawn chair by the pool, slathered in sun screen. That alone made me look healthier pretty quick. (I tan in a heart beat.) I think I had three massages from a short, stocky Mexican masseuse with hands like healing gloves and forearms of steel. I walked down the beach several times a day, just taking in each color and texture and flavor. The incredible turquoise of the water, sparkling like crystalline as it reflected off the sun and the waves, darkening as the water grew deeper. The many colors and texture variations of sand – from heavy, brown and wet to that out-of-reach of the waves – tan and loose and most exhausting to walk in. It reminded me of the sand gully back at home.

The smells that mingled in the air were usually some combination of sun screen, barbecue, pizza, French fries, any number of blossoming flowers, and the dampness that permeates everything within the tropics.

 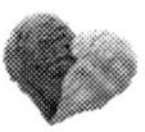

Of course, my issues with food didn't stay at home. Why would they? That little devil that I sometimes saw sitting on my shoulder was overjoyed at the fact that food was served predominately as a buffet. "Eat all you want! Whenever you want. You're on vacation," the devil would taunt me. From fast food to Mexican fare, to cakes and cookies, to a big bowl of granola and freshly cut fruit … there was something available to eat nearly 24/7. Usually something at least somewhat healthy could be found at each meal, if one looked hard enough. But I didn't want to work that hard.

The biggest blessing for me was that traditional Mexican pastries aren't covered with frosting as they are in the US. And that, combined with the constant humidity that left the cakes pretty spongey in a not-so-good way, (they tasted to me as though they'd accidentally fallen into a bathtub before being arranged on the dessert table. Yuck.) No need to worry about binging on those!

However, not to fear, little devil on my shoulder, the hotel gift shop kept a regularly stocked shelf full of Snickers, Twix, and Pay Days and a freezer full of Dove Bars, Drumsticks, and Popsicles. These weren't included in our all-inclusive hotel rate, but that didn't stop me. I still craved my sugar, my chocolate, my frosting. And much to my overwhelming glee, on my first trip to San Miguel to see which businesses were still open, I discovered that Hostess sold cupcakes there too! Thank you, Jesus, Mary, and Joseph! I loaded up a bag of them to take back to my room … figuring they would last a day or two. I knew I would need more trips to town to refill my stash throughout the week. Good thing the hotel was about eight miles out of town and I had no car.

I did go on a couple of SCUBA dives and, boy, did Miss Mojo get a wake-up call that had her ready to rock and roll suddenly, at least for a while.

I hadn't dove in several years so I asked the guy at the dive shop if it would be alright if I went out in the beginners' boat on my first trip, figuring no one would have high expectations of me that way. And the dive masters were actual instructors, as opposed to the guides who were just that – guides, meant to show capable and experienced divers great sights under the waves. Not to hold hands with newbies or the nervous.

While an instructor was more expensive, it felt worth it. To err on the safe side, I just paid for one dive, in case for some reason I just wasn't up for more. My instructor's name was Louis and he was a character. I told him about my limited experience and how it had been a long time since I'd donned my dive gear.

"No problema," he smiled an almost seductive smile at me – or was I making that up? I wasn't sure. It had been so long since I'd flirted with anyone that I really didn't know what it even looked like any more. "You just stay close to me, OK?" He winked at me, then returned to his task of readying everything for the half dozen people on the boat. I thought that staying close wouldn't be too tough … he was nearly gorgeous. About 5'9" (tall for Mexico), obviously fit. He wore a shortie wet suit, which exposed his extra muscular legs and arms, the top clinging to his tight body, leaving just enough wondering for my imagination. He had a full head of thick, black hair that was as unruly as was his salt and pepper mustache. Definitely an island guy.

I continued to watch him out of the corner of my eye as he interacted with all the other students; giving advice to

 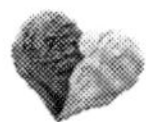

some, encouragement to others, and just laughter to those who he knew were scared to death.

With all final inspections complete, he jumped into the water where he put on his own gear, then instructed us to jump in, one by one, while he watched all the greenhorns fall like reluctant lemmings into the sea. The lemmings needed much hand-holding and he was very patient with each one, tightening a flipper here, adjusting a mask there, taking a couple of divers by the hand and pulling them along with him until they felt comfortable enough to go it alone. I was impressed. It takes a huge amount of patience to keep a bunch of newbies safe and comfortable even only in 35 feet of water. And he kept his smile up the whole time. Whether it was fake or genuine, it did the job of keeping everyone comfortable and feeling safe.

I kept within easy visual distance of him, rediscovering my sea legs quickly, much to my great happiness. When he would stop to help a student with one thing or another I would practice my buoyancy – the ability to hold yourself at a given spot in the water – very important so that you don't go crashing into the coral and damage it. Or, conversely, if you want to see some cool creature that was hiding under a ledge of coral, you would be able to hold your body steady in one place to watch it for a few moments.

I was enjoying getting my comfort level back and while waiting for Louis I practiced a few somersaults. I was having fun! The depression for that particular moment was gone as I became absorbed into the underwater world and its treasures.

The dive was great for me. Not for the usual excitements of underwater creatures and colorful corals, although those are usually my favorite part. But that dive was my first step in my new adventure. What came next was icing on the cake ...

The dive over, the captain pulled the boat up to the dock and everyone grabbed their gear and headed back to their hotel rooms to clean up. I'd had such a good time I asked Louis if I could go with the next group that was leaving in twenty minutes.

"Sure," he said. "So, it all came back to you, I see?" (Was he flirting with me again?)

"Yes, and easier than I thought." I was beaming. (I still didn't know what, if anything, I was supposed to do in response.)

"Just let me tell Pierre that you'll be joining his group, as I'm finished for the day."

Darn. I was disappointed to see him go. I had felt safe under his guidance. But he had assured me that I'd done great and I had to admit to feeling so as well. I heard him talking to Pierre about adding me to his group, and what he said next took my breath away ... he finished telling Pierre that I was a certified diver who just hadn't had her flippers wet in a while, then he said, "Don't worry about her – she's a mermaid."

Miss Mojo did back flips!

A mermaid? Me?

Here I was, shaking in my boots for so many months at home – feeling lost, and alone and certainly not capable of anything big, and just like that he recognized my abilities as someone quite competent and able to handle just about anything!

If this was a sign of things to come, I thought – bring it on!

***

 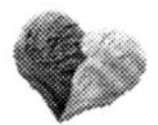

I found an incredible peace in Cozumel that vacation, which gave me hope. Actually, I suddenly felt a closeness to God that I had never experienced in my life. One night I sat all alone on the beach long into the wee hours of the night. Being away from civilization and all its lights the stars were especially intense and crystal clear. The full moon was enormous. The sound of the gentle waves lapping at the sand at my feet was almost deafening in the quiet. And in that quiet, I truly had an epiphany.

It's probably important to note here that, before this time, God and I weren't on the greatest of terms. Yes, I believed in God and had participated in all the church functions growing up, but I guess I had blamed God for some bad things that had happened in my life and I hadn't really gone out of my way to be friends with him. Yet out of nowhere I was startled by the most gentle voice. (Remember, I was all alone out there on the beach.) I truly believe that God connected with me at that moment.

His message was simple: He hadn't forgotten me. The devil didn't win. I wasn't being punished. All that had occurred to me had happened for a reason. They were life's lessons. And now it was time for me to heal. And when I was strong and healthy again, he had a job for me coming down the road.

I kept trying to make sense of what had occurred but there was no other explanation. I swear I was alone on that beach. And no – I hadn't been drinking. (Remember, I'd rather have my Hostess cupcake than alcohol. So nope – I wasn't under any influences unless chocolate has recently been discovered to have new hallucinogenic properties.)

The best analogy for what I went through during those moments is the commercial for M&M's Candies at Christmas where Santa Claus and the M&M characters suddenly find themselves face-to-face with each other and the M&M's say, "He is real!" at the same time that Santa says, "They are real!" And they all pass out on the floor in shock.

This was truly a turning point in my life.

I sensed that the overwhelming feeling of safety I'd felt in Cozumel was given to me for a reason. I also knew all too well that the gloom of winter in the States would only add to my stress. The many dark, snowy days sometimes made it hard for me just to get out of bed, much less function optimally. Considering that it was late November, I knew I could count on a lot of snowy, cold, and dreary months ahead. But now, with the added stress of a relationship in shambles, it felt nearly impossible to handle. That was already apparent with the suicidal thoughts I'd done battle with already. Maybe the next time I felt so low wouldn't end as well. I couldn't take that chance. It simply wouldn't be fair to Shaun. The Cozumel sunshine called to me like the mother of any newborn creature. I knew in my heart that my recovery would occur fastest in this new paradise where I felt right at home.

So, before my week was over I had lined up a job at the same hotel at which I'd been a guest. Then I flew home, packed my bags, and told my friends I was going to move to Cozumel for six months of healing. Everyone immediately thought I was crazy. At first, I was pretty sure that they simply didn't take me seriously. After all, it was going on Christmastime and everyone was getting wrapped up in their own holiday issues and, since I looked calmer, they felt that I was back on

 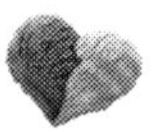

solid ground, I was OK again, and would simply get on with my life. Nothin' wrong with her! I think they were thinking, "Yeah, everyone says they're going to move to Paradise when they come home from someplace great. She'll get over it." But as I began to make plans to escape the winter at home, they finally started to believe me.

I tell people that I ran away from home that winter. Heck, since I never did that as a child, I was fully entitled to do so as a grown-up, wasn't I? My daughter was in college so I was past the responsibility of daily mothering. I had already filed for divorce and therefore had no one to be accountable to at home. My part-time job I knew I could replace with another upon my return. And I found folks to watch my house and care for my animals, surprisingly quite easily. It occurred to me that all those pieces had fallen into place for a reason.

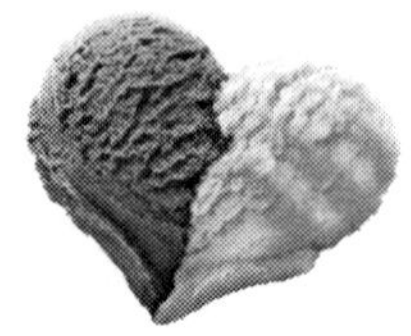

CHAPTER 8

Cozumel, My Cozumel

While my depression didn't just suddenly disappear, I could feel it shift a bit, almost immediately with the glorious sunshine feeding me daily and the distance away from the emotional situation at home making me feel so much less stressed. I loved watching CNN on cable TV every morning, and laughing at the horrible winter weather in Denver. It was the icing on the cake as I slipped into my shorts and sandals every day! I had no phone (until months later), no mail, no car, and no friends with me. I did email with my daughter a couple of times per week but that was back in the day that most people had to go to an Internet coffee house to email, where you paid like five bucks an hour to use their computers and get on the Net. So, emails were few and far between.

My life was very simple in Cozumel. I worked six days a week from about 8:30 a.m. to about 1 p.m., functioning as a concierge, although my real job was working for the hotel's time share company where they still sold vacation memberships to excited vacationers who got sucked into the romance of the island, just like I had. (They just couldn't hide out there for six months as I could.)

 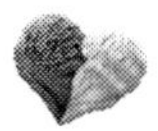

My concierge role had me acquainting guests to the layout of the hotel, to helping them line up their diving, to advising them on which shops in town would give them the best discounts, and just about anything else you could imagine. I even got requests for pot from some nurses from Texas but I hadn't a clue where to go for that! (Although it probably wouldn't have been too hard if I really felt the urge).

I rented a small, efficiency apartment for $500/month in a really nice part of town, right near a huge church. (It seemed like God still had me in his sights.) It came with cable TV, fridge, oven, and a maid three days a week who also washed and changed the linens. And all utilities were included! It was about a half dozen blocks from the downtown shops and plaza, and just a couple of blocks from the local grocery store, pretty similar to a small Walmart. Above all, I felt very safe there. It was perfect!

I walked everywhere that first month, learning my way around town. Unless I wanted to just sit home and watch TV all night, I figured exploring on foot was a good opportunity for learning as well as exercising. And despite the fact that I had discovered Mexico Hostess cupcakes, I started to shed some pounds with all the moving I was doing! And, as I would notice over time, as my happiness increased, my weight decreased. Interesting discovery, no? (Or as they oftentimes say in Cozumel; "Si. No?")

By month two, I had bought a bicycle and started extending my exploring even farther. Sometimes on my day off I would ride clear to the other side of the island where the surf was wild and dangerous, but intensely beautiful as it came pounding in from the Atlantic. I certainly burned some calories there – especially in the head wind that seemed to always be in my face, no matter which direction I was riding.

As for meals, I was thrilled that they had Cocoa Krispies cereal, one of my all time favorites. The milk wasn't anything to write home about – it was pretty much whole milk or nothing! (After drinking skim for years, that wasn't going to work.) So instead, I'd pour a bottle of strawberry liquid yogurt over my cereal and it truly hit the spot! For lunch, I got to eat at the hotel buffet as part of my job – taking hotel guests to lunch before the time share tour. So that was lucky. I made that my main meal for the day. And for dinner I'd often just stop in at a little local taco shop or street vendor's kiosk for a couple of tacos or maybe a burger. I gave up making meals entirely and my fridge only had liquid yogurt and diet soda in it.

While I still found solace in sugar, I quickly figured out that just like at home in Colorado, if I didn't bring junk food home, I didn't often eat it. If I suddenly had a craving for something sweet at 11 p.m., then I had to go out and find it. However, unlike in the States, most shops were closed by 9 p.m., so late night snacking was not easy – but that was the idea. No junk food could be kept in the house. Period.

Another weight loss activity I found helpful was kick-boxing. I had been taking kick-boxing classes at home prior to my Thanksgiving trip and had found it to be incredibly helpful in reducing stress and, as luck would have it, the local Mexican Walmart had punching bags and gloves for sale. After checking in with my landlady to see if she'd mind if I hung the bag on the back porch, (she lived a floor beneath me) she was thrilled with the idea and asked if I'd teach her as well.

 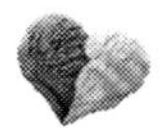

I loved taking my anger, frustration, and tears out on my punching bag. I even drew a pirate face on it so that he looked evil. Jab. Punch. Upper cut. Round kick. Back fist. Repeat ... Jab. Punch. Upper cut. Round kick. Back Fist. Repeat.

I went through the motions over and over with the sweat rolling off my forehead and into my eyes in the nearly 100 percent humidity, my eyes stinging and blurred until I would stop to wipe them dry with a towel. Then I added jump roping to my new routine, 1,000 skips per set. In a matter of just a couple of weeks of all this new eating and working out, the weight started melting off. And as the weight left, Miss Mojo began to feel a little stronger each day.

Although there were a few situations where my Mojo had a close call or two...

***

The first happened at work. The day the hotel hired me it was their responsibility to get all the proper paperwork squared away with the government. They had me sign a bunch of papers and I didn't give it a second thought, until a few months into my stay when some very serious people from immigration showed up at the hotel and they instantly got into it with my sales manager. Mind you, I speak no Spanish, so I was clueless about what was going on. But I was able to discern that it had something to do with me.

After several minutes of heated discussion, the serious folks left and my boss Ricardo headed over to me. He was a giant of a man, easily 250-plus pounds, but with the demeanor of a pussy cat and one of those slow to rile personalities.

"So, Mary Jo," he said. "I guess your paperwork got lost somehow and now immigration is unhappy."

"Is everything going to be OK?" I asked, getting a bit worried. He plopped down in a chair next to me, the chair straining to stay tall.

"Well, I think we'll be fine but immigration says that if you don't go to City Hall and fill out the proper forms within the hour, they will deport you."

I could feel the blood drain from my face. I had no idea if that meant I just had to go pack and depart right away or if they would be back in an hour with a police van to take me away in handcuffs, or what! Ricardo saw that I was in shock and likely to fall apart any second and in his most reassuring voice he said, "They have assured me that everything will be fine, but you must go now and get this taken care of immediately, OK?"

He patted my arm with his beefy hand and said, "Go. And take as much time as you need." He turned and lumbered away, returning to bigger matters than me.

Well, I did get the matter taken care of, although it took a bit of an ordeal to get it all handled as I didn't speak Spanish and the immigration people didn't speak any English. I ended up needing to take one of my work friends (Pierre from the dive shop) along to translate. Little did I know that he'd be such a talented translator as his mom was French, his dad Mexican, and he spoke fluent English as well.

I stood by as Pierre and the young Latina woman behind the counter went back and forth about various topics. I had no idea what she was asking of him until he'd repeat her question to me in English. What was my home address in the States?

 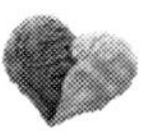

What was it in Cozumel? How long was I planning on staying, etc. Then finally they both acted puzzled and kept looking back and forth from my face to each other. Now what? I wondered.

Finally, Pierre asked me, “What color do you call your eyes?” Of the choices listed on the paper, I guess mine just didn’t fit with the typical Latin dark brown eyes. Mine are something of a hazel, but seemed to change with the lighting. They were stumped, until after much debate, they agreed to call them grey. And just like that, I was legal again – at least for another six months! Crisis averted.

One of my other Miss Mojo tests had to do with getting a Moped. While my move from walking to a bicycle was definitely an improvement, there were still some situations where biking wasn’t that great – like biking at night. I just didn’t do it. Which either meant I was back to walking or else taking a taxi. The idea of owning a moped sounded great in terms of practicality, but I’d never been as adventurous as to ride one before by myself.

Plus, the American consulate in Cozumel couldn’t say enough about just how dangerous moped riding was on the island. Apparently most of the injuries were caused by inexperienced riders who were on the island for the day and thought they’d make their own tour on the back of a cute, little red scooter. And, most commonly, they’d never ridden one before. Add to that the fact that Cozumel’s streets are alternating one-way, which takes a bit of getting used to, and the other fact that drivers were extremely aggressive (especially the taxi drivers) and the odds for injury shot up pretty quickly. And I surely didn’t want to end up in a hospital there as they were not prepared to handle much more than the simplest of first aid.

Still, I wanted one, despite the fact that my time there was whittling itself down quickly. I kept watching how the local people made a scooter into a multi-person carrier. I think the most people I saw on one Moped at one time was five! How, you ask? So, Daddy is the driver with his 3 year old standing up in front of him and between his legs, the 6 year old sitting behind Dad, and Mamma on the back holding the baby in one arm and with one hand around the poppa's middle. They thought nothing of it. To me, it was an accident waiting to happen.

There were other interesting Moped positions too ... for example, some of the more matronly ladies apparently weren't comfortable riding astride and would instead, keep their knees together and ride side saddle. (Now that took guts – or stupidity. I'm not sure which.)

One Moped image I got a kick out of was of a middle-aged woman zooming down the street – hair flying in the breeze – a look of determination on her face, and a dead chicken hanging upside down from one hand as she wove in and out of traffic, apparently headed home to throw him in the pot for dinner!

I only had three months to go before heading home. So, while common sense told me to leave a Moped alone I bought a nearly-dead one that indeed got me around until just about my last day on the island. Talk about a new freedom! I even got pretty darned good at navigating the many one-way streets and the crazy taxi drives. I could drive around to the far side of the island if I wanted, with the sun and wind on

 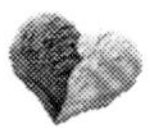

my face and the turquoise waves providing both the visual display and the sound track to go along with it.

I was heading into new, adventurous waters once again.

But there was one last test Miss Mojo faced that I didn't anticipate. Nor was I sure how it would play out when I found myself in the middle of it ...

***

I went jogging at times, once I started getting more fit. Most often along the waterfront and through the downtown streets, but occasionally I would venture off the main drag with all its fanciness. To the tourists who just visit for the day, most go home with an impression that Cozumel is just shops and day activities. But if one walks inland just a few blocks you'll quickly see how the real people live. There is no fanciness. Certainly no opulence. Many extended families live in tiny houses or apartments. Dogs frequently either run wild up and down the streets or are chained up or behind gates, attempting to look like a security system.

While I'd owned a couple of Old English sheep dogs when I was in college, I was pretty uncomfortable around dogs I didn't know, after having been badly bitten once as a kid. So I kept my radar up for any loose ones and usually the ones I did see out of a fenced space were usually conked out with the heat, and certainly not looking to spend any extra energy, at least not until things cooled off later in the day.

***

Except for this one day …

I was jogging along the back streets when two loose, moderately large dogs caught drift of me, apparently too close to their territory. They took to barking, very aggressively, and headed straight for me, full tilt.

My heart was in my throat. I knew I couldn't outrun them and the distance was closing fast. And I knew if they were as aggressive as they appeared to be, I could be one nasty mess in a matter of seconds. I did a quick look-round to see if I could get any help from any bystanders but no, no one in sight. My option and time were running out quick. My adrenaline was pumping full force and I could feel it coursing through my body, instantly driving my blood pressure and heart rate into overdrive. I felt a shiver race through me.

Suddenly, instead of running, I turned and faced the hungry canines and I began to bark at them in my most deadly, threatening, screamingly loud barks I could come up with. *"GRUFF, RUF, RUF, RUF,"* I barked. I waved my arms in the air over my head to make myself as big as possible. And I headed straight towards them, all the time keeping the barking going.

Apparently they hadn't run into this scenario before and they stopped dead in their tracks, likely thinking, "What the hell is that crazy thing?" I kept charging them, still barking as loud as possible. It felt like it was in slow motion but I'm sure it was only a matter of seconds when the once brave mutts turned tails and headed somewhere – anywhere – else, with only a quick look back once or twice to make sure I wasn't after them! They literally tucked tails and ran!

 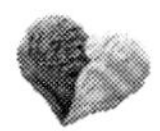

Catching my breath – I was panting like a racehorse and sweating to beat the band – from somewhere I could hear laughter. After running my hand across my brow to hopefully stop the sea of sweat and adrenaline pouring off my face, and letting my eyes refocus again, I realized that there were a couple of local workmen working on a house across the street. They had apparently seen the whole thing and were duly impressed. They started clapping, when they saw that I saw them there.

They waved and whistled and laughed for quite some time, giving me a thumb's up signal before they hopped in their truck and drove away, leaving me reassessing the whole ordeal in a little bit slower motion.

Holy crap! I just out-threatened two nasty looking canines who could have had me for lunch! I knew that, just a few weeks before, during my feel sorry for myself, depressed days, I certainly wouldn't have reacted the way I did.

There was a new me surfacing, and I was rather liking it. What's more, if Miss Mojo did back flips over being a mermaid, what the hell would she do after this?

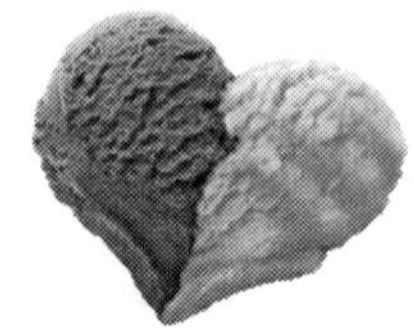

CHAPTER 9

Good Enough Love

Little did I know during my six months' stay on the island that so many of my experiences would lead me to a new profession when I got home – helping people with their relationships.

Hell, at that time I didn't even have a decent relationship with myself. But through my observations and many conversations with a wide variety of vacationing women, plus my own experiences experimenting with love, I developed quite a knowledge base that I would turn into several books over the coming years.

First, was the observation part where I saw so many unhappy vacationers each week. They were all thinking that a week in the sun would repair their bigger issues at home. (Hmmm ... sound familiar?) I watched husbands and fathers ignore their wives and kids completely. I saw wives walking six paces behind their men – as if they were lackeys, not loved ones.

I watched as one couple ate dinner and she never once was able to look him in the eye, much less carry on any kind of conversation, as he spent the entire meal berating her. (He was just loud enough to make sure that several tables of folks nearby would also hear his scolding.)

 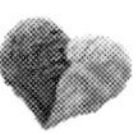

Then there was a couple who inquired about SCUBA lessons. I could tell that the wife (a very tiny gal) was terrified but went along with the plan because the husband (huge, linebacker-type guy) pressured her into doing it. I was going to be on their dive boat and when I got off work I headed to the dive shop to see how they were progressing and if they'd be OK to go out on the dive.

Unfortunately, the wife got scared after just a few moments under the water in the pool. She came up sputtering and terrified. Then, recognizing the anger and disappointment in her husband's face, started apologizing to him, to the dive instructor, and even to me, for chickening out on the dive. She was nearing a panic attack by then. She did, finally, convince the husband to go without her and, when things calmed down, she asked me if she could try it again the next day. I reassured her that it would likely be no problem, but I highly suggested that she do so without the grouchy husband along.

And guess what? She did fine! Without having the big galoot hanging over her every move. Criticizing. Chastising. Condemning. She mastered the "Intro to SCUBA" class and went out in the ocean with the mammoth man the next day, and had a successful dive.

Those were just a few of the observations that caught my eye, as I kept wondering what true love looked like. Did it look like that? Were people that lonely, that desperate for love, that they would accept good enough love, rather than great love?

Or was this not love at all?

I was still seeking the answer to that question.

Next came the conversations I had with so many women, in which I gleaned much. It would generally start with an American woman approaching me at my concierge desk for some sort of info, as they'd heard I spoke "good English." Then, once I answered their questions and they felt they knew me a little – perhaps over a few days – they would almost always end up asking me, "What are you doing here?" After all, I was living in a tropical paradise working for peanuts. Who does that?

My reply was always, "I'm running away from home and a divorce." At which point they would quickly pull up a chair and begin to tell me their story; middle-aged, empty nesters, unhappy with their marriage of 20-plus years, and trying to figure out what they were going to do with the rest of their lives. They were confused and frustrated just like me. And they all told me that they wished they had the guts to do something crazy like I had done.

I assured them, they too could do anything they put their minds to. But no, most of them were pretty stuck. Like hamsters on the wheel, they didn't know how to get off.

Most of these women were just desperately lonely – despite being in a relationship and having a mate. Rarely did they mention sex. For most of them, they needed to find themselves before they would feel comfortable getting naked with someone. Even with their husbands of many years.

There was one woman who did break that rule. I'll call her Kathy. She was very wealthy and had come to spend the entire winter at the hotel. Like me, she was running away from home and a divorce. She was in her 60's, very short, thin, and fashionable, but had a bad limp from a troublesome hip and

 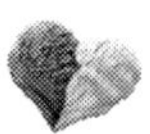

walked with a cane. She spent a lot of money on clothes. Hell, she spent a lot of money on everything. Throughout the season she brought various friends and family members to spend time with her at the hotel. Her grown twin girls for a week. Her parents for a week. Girlfriends, and others. She tipped well, thus everybody knew Kathy and everyone wanted to be her waiter.

I thought I'd gotten to know her pretty well until she shocked me one day when she approached me at my desk, looked both ways to make sure no one was near, and then, in her softest whisper, she said, "OK, I think I know you well enough by now to ask you this." She looked both ways again, to double-check that no one could overhear her.

Following her lead, I too checked both directions for any high-surveillance equipment or spies who might see us talking together. God knew what was coming.

"I need a man (slight pause, as if she had trouble getting it out), and I'm not kidding. Can you get me one?" She winked at me, with a "You get my drift" sorta message implied.

That wasn't what I was anticipating. I took it she was implying that she wanted a gigolo and was hoping that in my role as concierge, I would know how to procure said man.

I could tell she was near to tears. She must have been feeling pretty low to have to ask me for help with her problem. And I'm sure the look of shock on my face didn't help her any.

It took me a minute to find my voice. "Let me get this straight," I started, "you want a man for s…."

"Yes," she interrupted me. "For s-e-x," she spelled it out. "I'm not thinking I'd get lucky enough to find love. But I'd be satisfied just to have some amazing sex with some young pup before I die." The look on her face was absolutely serious, as she awaited my reply.

I was stumped on that one. I thought the requests for pot were brazen enough, but this? This would take some research. I told her to give me to day to look into it.

I then promptly tracked down one of my co-workers who had been the manager at Carlos and Charlie's busy saloon for quite some time. If anyone would know about such things, Pato would. So I approached him, quite uncertain how to ask.

"Hey Pato," my voice was tentative. He looked up from his card game where several of the timeshare employees hung out awaiting their next couple to tour the property.

"Hmmm?" he replied.

"You know that lady, Kathy? She's been here all winter? She's really wealthy?" I held my breath, rather hoping he didn't know her and I could simply cut my duties and run.

"Yeah, everybody knows her," he replied. Probably wondering what on Earth that had to do with him.

I cleared my throat as I tried to appear cool but he could readily sense that I wasn't. He looked like he wanted to say, "Get it out, girl," but he held his tongue.

"Well …" I started, "she just told me she needs a man and she's not kidding. Can you find her one?" I could feel my face go red as he suddenly got the picture and laughed out loud.

When at long last he finished his chuckling he asked, "So how much does she pay?" As if he had this conversation with people every day. "She's old," he explained.

I never saw that one coming either! Jeez! How naive was I? I think I made his whole day as he waited for my next mumbling. "I don't know how much she pays!" I tried to act

 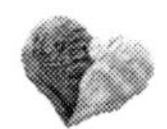

tough. Or at least not stupid. He was enjoying every minute of this, I realized. I, on the other hand, just wished it were over.

He scratched his head as if deep in thought, then finally came up with an idea.

"Go ask Juan. He always needs money." He was barely able to contain himself, I was sure, at my stupidity. Holding his hand over his mouth by then, attempting to hide his laughter.

"OK, thanks." I said, and moved on as quickly as possible before Pato could come unglued and announce the story out loud to everyone.

So I actually went to find Juan, who was on the opposite side of the room, reading some paperback to fill the time. He was Kathy's match in terms of size. About 5 foot 4 inches, one hundred twenty five pounds of slender muscle. With soft curly hair and a small mustache that made him look a bit sinister, although he wasn't in the least. He was, however, a player and was often into gambling, drinking, and partying. He was also a widower, having lost his wife in a drowning accident on the other side of the island years before. And was a single dad of a 12-year-old son.

Once again I mustered up my nerve. After clearing my throat, and Juan looking up at the sound, I used the same line. "Hey Juan, you know that lady, Kathy, she's been here all winter … ?"

Not seeing that this conversation would likely have anything exciting to do with him, he simply said, "Yeah, what of it?" and returned to his book.

I cleared my throat again and said, "She just told me she needs a man and she's not kidding. She asked me if I knew anyone who might fit the bill and Pato suggested I speak to you."

As the concept became clear in his mind, he sat bolt upright, closed the book, and dropped it on the table. I could tell he was a good possibility, then he suddenly said, "How much does she pay?"

I couldn't believe my ears! Were these guys for real?

"I don't know," I replied once again. Hoping this nightmare would come to an end and I'd wake up from this craziness soon.

"Well, where is she?" He was on the hunt. I told him that I'd just recently seen her at the pool. And off he went.

The long and the short of this story is that Kathy and Juan did fall in love and ended up together for quite some time. She moved in with him on the island for several months each year. She bought him a car and paid for his son's education. She even invited him to live with her in the States but he wouldn't leave his island home. For Kathy, her time with Juan was a time that stopped her loneliness, and whether their relationship lasted two months or two years, it brought huge happiness to her life.

***

Unlike Kathy, who never had to worry about her weight, many women struggle with their weight when their relationship status changes. I know when I'm seeking a man I'm much more aware of what I eat and how I take care of my body. I don't want to get naked with someone if I don't feel happy with my self.

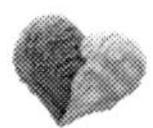

Conversely, when I'm head over heels in love, my mind doesn't crave all the junk it usually does normally. I don't need to fill that emptiness that goes along with being lonely or alone with sugar and junk.

And there is one other possibility about weight and relationships ... some women watch their weight during the courting and early relationship stages but then once their relationship is solid (through marriage or something else) they quit caring for their bodies anymore. And as time goes on, the weight goes up. I suspect that they are still using food to stuff an emptiness they still haven't filled. And in most situations, until that emptiness is discovered and addressed, through therapy and other methods, their battle with weight can likely follow them for a lifetime. These issues were beginning to intrigue me.

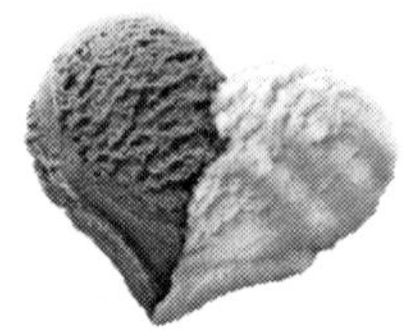

CHAPTER 10

Love Or Lust?

Yes, indeed, I fell in love with Cozumel.

And I fell in love *in* Cozumel, with a man!

I really hadn't been man-shopping. Hell, I didn't even know how to man shop, or date, or as I mentioned before, even flirt! I'd been off the market for 25 years and being in the middle of a tough divorce did not leave me seeking male companionship. And although I loved my little apartment and my freedom to only be responsible for me, I still went home to an empty house at the end of the day while most of my new friends went home to their families and loved ones.

That was the biggest shock of the entire divorce process ... in some ways I just felt like I'd left one uncomfortable situation and replaced it with another. So I ended up spending most evenings hanging around downtown, watching the tourists, shopping the little family-run stores for silver jewelry that I loved. (It was cheap and there were thousands of items to choose from.) I got to know many of the shop keepers and their families personally and even now when I go to Cozumel for an easy get-away with friends, I'll hear someone shout my name as I walk through the many shops.

"Mary Jo Fay," they will yell, as they run over to give me a big hug. Of course, the friends I travel with are usually quite shocked that so many folks seem to know me, but I remind them that at 5 foot 8 inches tall and with short, spikey blonde hair like I have, I stand out in the crowd and am a bit hard to forget.

One night Kathy and I agreed to have dinner in town and headed for one of the small places that had only one table occupied when we arrived. As we stepped up to the entrance we were met by an attractive Mexican man who made much of us as he directed us to the tropical center of the building filled with bamboo, flowers of all colors, and a bubbling fountain. It was like a small jungle within the inside of the restaurant. Quite charming.

"Good evening, Señoritas," he flattered us, for at our age we should be labeled Señoras.

"My name is José and let me welcome you to Pepe's!" He pulled each of our chairs back, then settled them in under us as we found the right spot. "And what may I call you beautiful ladies this evening,?" he inquired.

"I'm Mary Jo and this is Kathy," I answered. We knew that with only one occupied table besides us he'd stand on his head to serve us tonight. His tips would depend on just how good his performance was, and he knew it.

"And where are you lovely ladies from?" (I had to admit that his smile did look genuine. Plus, he was about my height, had a strong body, handsome face, nicely cut hair, was likely about ten years younger than me, and oh yes – he had those amazing, muscular forearms that made me go gaga.)

Kathy answered this time, "I'm from Minnesota and MJ here is from Colorado." I could tell that she was enjoying his attentions as well, although she had her own groupies at the hotel who fought over her daily, since they knew exactly just how well she tipped. Then of course, she had Juan, but she had taken this night to hang with me. She was always looking out for men for me, she would do her best, I knew, to get him interested in me.

He was very animated, spoke excellent English, and had mastered politeness to a T.

"And what can I get you ladies to drink?" he awaited our answers, note pad at the ready.

"I'll have a margarita, no salt," Kathy said, starting us off.

"And you, Señorita?" he beamed at me. You couldn't get a much bigger smile than that.

"Coca Light, por favor," I replied, using the Spanish name for what we Americans call Diet Coke.

José grimaced, a bit of his effervescence going flat. "Oh, Señorita Maria José" (Spanish for my Mary Jo introduction). "You had to choose the one thing we don't have. I am so sorry, is there something else I could bring you?" (I could see the disappointment in his face, as he was likely calculating just how that may impact his tip.)

I said I'd be fine with water and off he went, rather dejected looking.

Kathy and I spent the next several minutes while he was gone commenting on his winning features. He was one of the handsomest men we'd run into, and I especially liked the tall part, since most of the men had Mayan roots, leaving them lucky to grow to 5 foot 5 or so.

Several minutes later, as we were giggling ourselves silly envisioning what other parts of his body might be like, a

 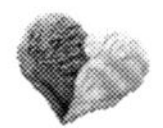

young bus boy arrived at our table, bringing Kathy's margarita and my Diet Coke! What the heck? We gave each other a look and attempted to ask the boy about it but it soon became clear that he didn't speak a word of English.

When José returned to take our order, I asked, "So I thought you didn't have any Coca Light? I'm confused."

Kathy and I were intrigued by now.

He smiled again, this time a bit mischievously, "We don't, but I paid the boy to run down to the little shop at the end of the block and pick some up just for you."

His tip just multiplied itself by ten! And he knew it.

And that's how the evening went. José bringing us endless chips and salsa, our main meal, extra guacamole, more Coca Light, and even gave us a free dessert, all the while keeping Kathy's glass full of margaritas. We must have been there for at least three hours, with him asking questions about Denver (*How about those Broncos?*) and Minnesota, then entertaining us with stories of his own. Neither Kathy nor I had laughed so much in ages. By midnight, the cook had gone home and the bus boy had finished picking up and cleaning everything for the next day. We knew we needed to say good-bye. But we knew where he worked now. We'd definitely be back! And Kathy and I would have much to talk about the next day back at the hotel.

We both gave José a huge bear hug, thanked him profusely for a wonderful evening, and left him with a $30 tip for our $30 meal! Not bad.

Kathy hailed a taxi to take her back to the hotel, and they dropped me off at my apartment on the way. I gave her a hug as well and sent her home, knowing that it would be hard to fall asleep after such an evening.

The next day was my day off and I was eager to see if I could run into José again. I had hardly been able to sleep all night, my mind and hormones had been racing. It had been so long since I had had feelings like I was experiencing. They left me excited as well as scared to death – simultaneously. On the one hand, I desperately craved human touch of the male variety. On the other hand, I really wasn't ready for any man to touch me, with the emotional confusion I'd been dealing with at home.

Of course, even 25 years ago when I had been dating, things were different. The rules had now changed and I didn't even know what the current rules were. Plus, my dating life when I was in my early twenties had been short and sweet. I'd had only a couple of boyfriends before I met Kevin and we'd gotten married. So even back then I was pretty inexperienced. There was just so much I didn't know I didn't know.

Then, of course, there was *my body*. I weighed somewhere in the 160's and didn't feel very ready too show it off to anyone just yet. At least I had been walking and biking and leaving some of those pounds behind. This just gave me more incentive to push it up a bit. So that day I grabbed my bicycle intending to go for a long ride but instead headed the few blocks into town to José's restaurant first. And as luck would have it, he was walking in that direction when I ran into him.

"Preciosa," he grinned, "how are you today?" He still looked delicious in his form-fitting black slacks and shirt – the uniform of his restaurant.

"I'm good, José, but what is preciosa?" I stepped off my bike and leaned on it for support, still a bit uncertain about what to do next. I wanted him to know that I liked him and I thought he liked me, but I didn't want him to think I would be jumping into bed with him overnight. How did one convey that, I wondered?

"It means, beautiful, because you are." (There was that flirting again. He definitely knew how to get a woman's attention. I mean, what woman *didn't* want to hear those kind of words from a cute guy?) He couldn't talk long as he was heading to work, but we agreed to have drinks after he got off work late that night.

Little did I know that simple evening would turn into the biggest whirlwind romance of my life…

Whether it was love or lust is hard to say. Because I certainly thought I was terrified of the whole idea of intimacy, but in his arms I felt safe and loved and desired. He never rushed me, always waiting for me to show my readiness for each next step until we reached the point that we couldn't keep our hands off of each other.

And everything I have ever heard about Latin lovers was true. His passion was endless. His touch lit my body on fire. His kisses were slow and patient. His tongue was amazing, exploring my neck, my ears, and oh, so many other places. He would tease me, toying with me for hours. Building up my excitement, then making me wait until I thought I'd go crazy.

He wanted me to teach him everything about my body and I was a bit nervous about that. But slowly he convinced me that he truly did want to know all the details of what made me tick and we would spend hours in bed talking about things we both liked or didn't like. The things we craved. The details of everything. And then we'd try them out on each other, over and over!

I loved his body. His weight was perfect, although he wasn't a gym rat. His ribs were just slightly visible through his skin and his muscles, in any variety of places, were firm and well shaped. His pectoral muscles were well defined. His stomach, flat. His chest hair incredibly sexy. And of course, I loved his chiseled forearms: muscular, with just the right amount of hair.

I had never been so open with someone about my body, nor been with someone who was so willing to teach me about his. He said the same about me.

I have to say that Miss Mojo was experiencing each moment right along with me, cheerleading from the side lines! And boy, was she getting stronger each day with all she was experiencing.

I could feel my strength returning. Was it purely a sexual release or perhaps it was being able to trust someone with my body. Wow! I couldn't think of the last time I had been so happy or so comfortable in the bedroom.

We spent every spare moment with each other. And it became a long-standing joke that I would say, in my most serious voice, "Now, José, no more sex today!"

And he would say, "We will see ..." and odds were, we'd find ourselves back in bed again. Although we did have to come up for air from time to time, at least for food.

He called me the love of his life. And told everyone so.

Sometimes, we'd take my Moped to the other side of the island, with him driving and me with my arms around his slim waist, feeling his body against my breasts. Those were days I was certain I'd died and gone to heaven. His body so close to mine for nearly an hour. The sea breeze and sun in our faces. The sky huge and blue and cloudless. I took in his scent and got lightheaded. In those moments, who thought about food? Not I!

Again I noticed how I no longer was craving my favorite junk foods during this time. In fact, most of the time we ate only one meal per day. We just didn't seem that hungry. I was getting more and more comfortable with my body as it shed the extra pounds. And he made me feel comfortable whether I lost those pounds or not.

We both had jobs to go to, so our hours together weren't unlimited, but we made the most of what we had. We spent many days on the beach. Snorkeled some. Danced some at one of the local dance spots or another. (He was a fabulous dancer.) It didn't matter what we did, as long as we were together.

One day we drove the Moped out to the small ruins on the island, admiring the remains of the Aztec people who lived there hundreds of years ago. On the way home, we came across a couple of senior citizen couples who had thought that renting Mopeds for the day would be a good idea and while they had made it all the way around the island without incident, 15 minutes from the Moped rental office they took a bad spill at a busy intersection.

It wasn't bad enough that they needed an ambulance, but the one woman was pretty upset and had several scratches that needed to be cleaned up. The nurse in me jumped into action and I took her to the grocery store nearby and got her cleaned up, as best I could.

She had been driving solo on her Moped but after the accident was scared to drive it the rest of the way back. So, José offered to drive her and I'd follow on my moped. Once there, he used his best PR skills to convince the Moped rental guy that the damage they'd caused to the bike really wasn't that bad, saving the couple a few hundred bucks they would likely have had to pay without his bargaining skills.

The lady I'd cared for asked me if that "cute New York fire fighter" was my husband. I didn't know what she was talking about, but then it occurred to me that he was wearing a t-shirt that said NYFD on it; apparently a shirt that a tourist had traded him for something else at one time or another. She was so impressed at how he had helped them and gave him twenty bucks for his effort.

It was things like that I will always remember about him.

Sadly, my time to go home grew near and we couldn't believe how quickly the time had passed. I'd promised my family who were watching out for my pets and property that I'd be back in six months and I couldn't let them down. I knew I'd asked a lot of them already.

We cried our eyes out at the airport, promising that we'd somehow make it work, long distance. But knowing in our hearts that it wouldn't pan out. Anyone knows who has ever been in that spot – it's way too difficult.

I did get back to see him, making a couple of trips for a week here and there but the chemistry had changed. That part of my life was just over. And over the following years I did date some other men who taught me much about relationships and love as well, but I credit José for getting me to drop my guard and let love in again.

The lessons learned in Cozumel actually would serve me for years to come. It had been my sanctuary while I healed. Now it was time to move on, start the next part of my life, whatever that might be.

Going back to civilization was hard but I have to admit that being close to family and friends did feel really good. And Miss Mojo and I had developed a new strength – badly needed strength, as I was once again going to be making some big changes.

***

The first thing I did was put the house on the market. That was tough. I'd spent 16 years there, had made many memories there. It had been the dream I'd had for years. Suddenly it was different. Now it was just a house, not a home anymore. I also sold the last two horses, which actually broke my heart more. I just knew I couldn't keep up a place that size any more. Not by myself.

I was in transition, not knowing what the next journey would be. And so after the house sold (and that took nearly a year), I sought out a temporary living arrangement to keep myself flexible. I ended up in a roommate situation in the mountains just west of Denver. The guy who owned the house, Patrick, was gone 90 percent of the time. He got on a plane every Monday morning and returned every Friday night. And if it was snow skiing season, he left the house Saturday morning to go work on ski patrol, then returned Sunday late afternoon, paid his bills, did his laundry, and packed to leave again the next morning.

It was a perfect situation for both of us. He got rent and I got a house essentially to myself. I only mention this brief living situation because it was where I gained back so much of my weight. And looking back at it, I have to laugh. It was truly one of my greatest excuses of all the great excuses I've used over the years.

Since Patrick and I were nothing more than roommates, that also meant we bought our own food as well. However, since the grocery store was a good 20 minutes each way, it was considered fair game to borrow something from each other, then replace it the next time either of us went shopping.

Living alone like I was, food did its great job of being a filler of emptiness, as always. And so, when my hunger (stomach or emotional) started working its way with me, I'd start searching first, through my stuff, seeking something sweet and satisfying. Because I refused to buy any junk in bulk to bring home, I was usually pretty good about not going overboard too often. I'd buy whatever junk I could when I went to town, something yummy at the bakery perhaps, then eat it in the car on the way home. (Yep, I never quit that habit, even after 7-Eleven!)

However, on nights when a good snow storm had settled over the house and I couldn't get out to procure my fix, I would start searching through Patrick's goodies. Mind you, he was about 5 foot 10 inches tall and not an ounce of fat on him. Ate healthy all the time too. But he did like an occasional Klondike bar. It didn't take me long to find his stash and I took the first one, thinking he'd understand if one was missing. It wouldn't be that big a deal. So, I'd eat one, despite the fact that ice cream bars really weren't on my favorites list. I gobbled it up right quick. Hmmmm ... I thought. Not so bad after all. I even licked the stick until the last traces of chocolate were gone.

Well, I said to myself, maybe just this one time, I'll allow myself two. Surely I'll have time to get to the store before he

 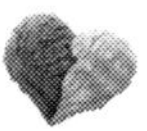

comes home and I can refill his supply. He'll never know the difference.

Made perfect sense to me. But that was before I realized that I would be house bound due to the snow for two and a half days. The Klondike bars barely made it past the first night.

By the time Patrick was due home, I'd been to the store and back and reloaded the freezer, just as he'd left it. I even pushed the wrappers to the bottom of the trash can to hide the evidence. It worked! He never knew a thing. And I – well, now I had a Plan B in the event of another snow-in. Which of course happens quite often in the mountains.

My "Plan C" came quickly on the tails of Plan B. Only this time it was one of those tubs of ready-made cake icing. I couldn't for the life of me understand why he would have cake icing on the shelf. He certainly didn't bake and he certainly wasn't a sugar junkie. The Klondikes seemed to be his only weakness and even those he only ate on a rare occasion.

And so one night, when I'd either already wiped out the Klondike supply or had gotten bored with them, I did it; I broke into the frosting! Just me, a spoon, and Pillsbury's Best Chocolate Frosting. What else could any God-fearing sugar junkie need? So, for the next 24 hours, I gorged on that stuff.

Then, of course I had to replace it, in case he might miss that little goodie on his pantry shelf next time he was home. I didn't find out until much later that it wasn't even his! It had been left there months before by an earlier roommate. So I'd gone through all those antics for nothing!

As it turned out, I was only there for about five months. He ended up meeting some gal and despite the fact he was barely ever home, she wasn't too keen on me being there, roommate or not!

It was time for me to go. All those Klondike bars and the Pillsbury's Best Frosting had landed me at 185 pounds!

Yep, the evidence was clear; whether I had no love or no lust, I always turned to my reliable standby, food, as my no kiss-and-tell lover.

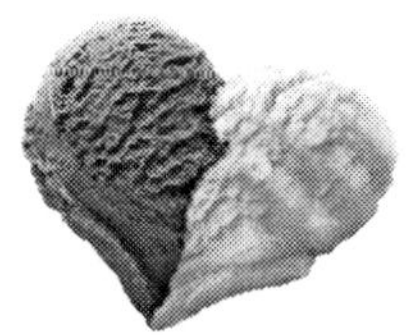

CHAPTER 11

Reality Check

My next adventure – another mountain "adventure" – began a few months later, in the spring of 2008. I'd been renting an amazing mother-in-law's apartment in the lower level of a big estate in the mountains just a few miles west of Denver, owned by a world-renowned musician with a world full of problems. In fact, if you looked up the word "narcissist" in the dictionary, you'd likely find his photo in lieu of a definition. He'd been a big deal in his younger years, when he was 18 or so. Played across the globe. Won some big international competition in Germany, even at his young age. Had been revered by thousands. But drugs and alcohol, as they usually do, took their toll and he'd dropped into the vacuum of great unknowns. All the while he thought he was still a big "known."

When I first moved in, he and his wife were separated and she lived in the place by herself and I think she was grateful to have someone around. She was friendly but kept pretty much to herself. It was perfect. I actually worked on two books during the ten months I lived there.

The place was incredible. It was situated on thirty acres of ancient pine forest with a half-mile-long (paved) driveway just to reach the house. It was a million dollar property, and I think the wife struggled to afford it during that time. There were no neighbors in sight except the guy who rented a loft apartment over the barn. I never saw him. The house itself was a sprawling ranch with a lower level that was a walk-out. That was where I lived. The owner occupied the main floor.

The whole place was decorated in Southwestern art, which I felt right at home with. Heavy Native American rugs. Cowboy and bronze horse statuettes. Dark, warm tapestry. There was even a photo of my landlord standing next to Ronald Reagan. (I told you – he'd really been somebody once upon a time.)

My living room was filled with sun for much of each day and drew visitors of many species to the windows and my door, when I left it open on nice days. The herd of elk that claimed the area as home numbered about 30. Some mornings I'd open up my outer door to find most of those 30 cows and their babies munching clover on my lawn. Some lying down. Some even watching me through my window. All looking curious but none looking very worried. They'd lived there for a long time apparently. And their only danger was that once a year during hunting season, the owners would shoot one or two for meat to last all winter. So other than the one or two unlucky ones who turned up on someone's plate, grilled to perfection, the elk were a contented herd in the yard.

They were amazing to watch, being so close. The females have a face only a mother could love, but the babies were so much fun to watch, with their antics during play and their snow-white spots to keep them camouflaged.

I learned a lot about elk during the time I was there. The young bucks were interesting and sometimes laughable. At

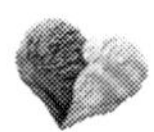

their young adult age, it was like they were living in limbo, with antlers just sprouting. Antlers are amazing. They are covered in sensitive tissue filled with blood that helps them grow. It would be a few years before those young males would look anything like the big bulls with their 6- or 8-point antlers, fighting each other, sometimes ferociously, with those weapons to win a mate. Or in the case of elk, a harem.

Aside from the elk, bears and mountain lions also shared the land. Although I never came face to face with one myself, I was driving up the driveway one night and a lion leaped across the road just ahead of me, his distinctive tail propelling him at top speed to avoid me. That took my breath away and I was always very cautious whenever I was out walking my dog on the property after that.

One reason I loved that place was that I was welcome to use the outdoor hot tub on the upper deck and, since the owners were rarely home, I had it all to myself. Being that far away from the city made star gazing that much better in the crisp, black sky. I was dating at the time and it was nice being able to share those moments with my gentleman, in addition to having a buddy for strolling through the grounds to walk my dog, always cognizant of those lions and tigers and bears … Oh, my!

My weight at this time was about 185 pounds. And while I could hang around the house and even go to the grocery store or other informal activities wearing my standby leggings and baggy sweaters, I had to dress up at least twice a month for my role as facilitator of an organization I called Denver's Best Dating, Mating, and Relating Meetup Group.

If you're not familiar with Meetup.com, it's an Internet company that helps connect folks who have similar interests.

Anyone can create a Meetup group. There are groups for single moms, hikers, bikers, investors, political supporters, and even people who like poodles. The topics are endless and just as with Facebook, this Internet app has spread like wildfire across the land.

My group was focused on helping singles ages 45 and up, bringing them together not only to meet other eligible daters, but to learn about navigating the tricky path of dating in today's world, especially for middle agers. At first I was a speaker at this group when a gal friend of mine ran it as a relationship book club. By that point I had already authored 3 books, based in part on my education in Cozumel, my own dating experiences, plus numerous stories of people I had met along my journey who were also struggling to find love. The friend had me join in as a guest author at a couple of her monthly events, neither of us knowing at that point in time I would eventually take over the group, ax the book club part, and run it for nearly ten years. I learned early-on that many of the people who came simply wanted to interact with each other, with only facilitation from me. They really didn't want to be lectured to. And they really didn't want to read books!

The group had a unique format, mixing men and women at small tables around the room where they got to share their own experiences with each other. They asked questions of the others within their group, bantering back and forth for the two-hour event. They told their own stories of success or failure in the love department. They picked each other's brains about who should do what when. (Who should call after the first date? Who should pay for the first date? That kind of thing.) And always I provided a specific topic for them to

share their thoughts over as well. At that time we had about 50 participants who came out twice per month. (Although the membership was well over 3,000!) People were not only meeting each other, many folks would linger at our venue for hours after the meeting came to an end! They were pairing off as the sparks flew!

Eventually for the lucky ones, marriage came next! I ended up getting my credentials to marry people in Colorado and, in fact, married 4 couples that I know of were from the group. In addition there were many others who lived together for years! It was so rewarding to see people find love with my little group. I had become a dating expert and people began signing up with me for dating coaching.

I created one other Meetup group called The Intimacy College, where I used my nursing background to teach men about women in the bedroom, and women about themselves. (Because so many women really don't know much about their own bodies! And if I could get both sexes to understand women and sex, we'd be 80% of the way towards great sex. Why? Because men simply need a place to have sex. Women need a *reason*!)

This was a lecture format where for 3 hours I talked about the tricky topic of intimacy because, believe it or not, even despite the ready availability of porn sites on the web, and our letting go of so many puritanical beliefs and behaviors in our culture, there was and is so much misunderstanding around sex that it's honestly amazing that anyone is having any satisfying sex at all! After the class, I would send them all home with a copy of my book, *Please Dear, Not Tonight: The Truth About Women and Sex*, and I was quite pleased to often get emails from my clients who had tried out some of the skills I had taught them in class and were happy to report success!

About the time the dating and intimacy business was growing nicely, I was also starting to coach folks with a completely different set of problems: they were enmeshed in a relationship (romantic or otherwise) with a narcissist and didn't know what to do about it.

How did I fall into that role? Well, another of my books, *When Your Perfect Partner Goes Perfectly Wrong*, focused on abusive, narcissistic people and how to recognize them and their behaviors … and how to steer clear of getting sucked into any kind of relationship with them to begin with. Some of my readers were desperately seeking information on how to get out of a toxic relationship after suddenly realizing they were definitely not in a healthy situation, but just didn't know there was a name for it … and things you could do about it.

If you're like many folks, you're likely not familiar with narcissism and narcissists either. Or perhaps you have thought that someone with this label simply has a big ego – and you would be partially right. But narcissists are more than just that. In their darkest form, they can be downright dangerous. (Most murder/suicides and other terrible behaviors involve extremely narcissistic people.)

After publishing that book and announcing my services online, people were calling me left and right about their unhealthy situations. Although not a therapist, I was a survivor of many narcissistic relationships in my own life and people begged to consult with me. I suddenly became a guru on the subject, as very little had been written about this destructive personality disorder at the time ... especially from the victim's

 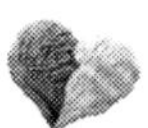

side of things. People just wanted to talk to someone who understood their situation. Most had no clue what to do. Should they stay in their stressful, anxiety-filled relationship or should they go? In many of the situations some didn't have a dime to their name. Their narcissistic mate was in control of all finances, among other things. If they left, they could be out on the streets starving, possibly with their children in tow.

Narcissistic people can be men or women. (Although more commonly men.) Young or old. Educated or not. Attractive or not. Wealthy or not. But their behavior is frequently controlling, manipulative, cunning, abusive, charismatic, charming, and sometimes deadly.

Their abuse can be physical; the visible bruising, broken bones, and more at least leaves evidence of their behavior. But more frightening is the non-visible abuse that goes on behind closed doors. Sexual. Emotional. Verbal. A constant berating, chipping away at any self-esteem that might still be barely hanging on by a thread. Then, there are things rarely seen by those outside the family. The wounds that often are deeper than any broken arm or black eye could ever be: the constant put-downs, verbal attacks, name-calling, threats, and so much more.

One of my clients told me the most horrid story of verbal and emotional abuse I'd ever heard of ... each morning her husband would say, "Jamie, what are you worth? And don't get it wrong or there will be hell to pay."

Each day, Jamie (not her real name) had to say, "I'm worth 29 cents, Honey. The price of a bullet!" Can you imagine?

One woman narcissist I knew personally would frequently tell her grown daughter, "I wish I would have had an abortion instead of having you." She had no qualms about speaking such horrible words right in front of her young grand daughter either. Talk about teaching our children by example. These are only a couple of examples of the hundreds of real-life stories people sent me. And these were the mild ones. One of the more dangerous ones was a man who locked his wife in the closet for 11 hours, forcing her to sit there with his gun in her mouth! Believe me, I couldn't make this stuff up.

Little did I envision becoming a consultant to folks about these very toxic people and their mates. It actually became a huge part of my life. I even had clients call me from as far away as the Middle East, Australia, and Europe. Narcissism knows no boundaries. And especially in the Middle East, where women are barely recognized as people, you can only imagine how narcissism runs rampant.

It was very difficult to work with the victims of narcissism for so many of them are so emotionally spent that they are afraid of their own shadows and carry a huge amount of negative energy that spreads to others. Most know they should leave their unhealthy relationships but fear the consequences. Some are too afraid to step outside their doors. Others swear that they really love this abusive person, believing that he (or she) really doesn't "*mean*" to abuse them. How he's promised it will never happen again. And of course, it does. But many of them are moms and are scared to death that their mate will take the children. And those threats are pretty powerful.

I was pleased that I did make a difference in some of their lives. I used many of their stories in a second edition of my book, which helped many of the victims feel as though their

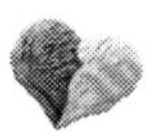

struggles had meant something. And every now and then I hear from successful past victims who have claimed their lives and their power back and are on the way to finding healthy love at last.

Anyway, getting back to weight ... you see now why I couldn't live in my leggings all the time. Which meant, with my weight climbing back up yet again, I had to go out and buy clothes that fit, to wear to these events. Not only do I hate shopping on good days, I really hate it when I have to buy bigger sizes. Damn those buttons and zippers that kept making me miserable. Sometimes I'd just not button or zip them and instead wore a belt that could be buckled in place (despite me not buttoning them) and still keep things where they should be. Sometimes I would buy those little extender things that would give both sides of my waistband just a little longer reach to get to the other side. It was looking like size 16 was on my doorstep. And I wasn't happy about it. Still, I kept eating like there was no tomorrow, yet always hopeful of a different outcome. (What was that definition of insanity again?) Duh.

On the bright side, I loved staying at that wonderful mountain respite I got to call home for nearly a year. I hated to leave it. It had been such a great creative space for me, helping me write 2 new books. But eventually the owners reconciled and the musician moved back home and that's when things got weird and I knew my time was up.

And I was on to the next adventure.

***

This time, I rented a condo in Aurora (a suburb of Denver) about five minutes away from Mom and my big sister, Barb, to our mother's great happiness. She was in her 80's and felt more safe with all of us close by. While I missed the mountains, since my creative juices flowed there, I did appreciate the availability and access of things in the city, including a 24 Hour Fitness just a few blocks away. Alarmed by the size 16s encroaching and desperately trying to keep my boundary strong there, so as not to let my muffin top get out of control – which it was definitely threatening to do, one day I told myself: "Enough is enough!" and I joined a fitness club!

Little did I know when I signed on the dotted line that I would end up spending seven years there in various stages of working out, playing, making new friends, and enjoying some happy times. When I joined, the membership kid told me that with my new membership I got a free workout assessment with one of their trainers, *would I be interested?* Sounded like a deal to me, so I told him to sign me up.

And within a couple of days I met the face of a young pup named Cody, who would come to change my life. Early 20-something. Body-builder competitor. Trainer. Handsome, and knew it. He had dark, wavy hair and eyes that smiled and sparkled. Plus a personality that was full as the dickens. You could see every muscle on his body. His calves, for example, were even more shapely than mine, and that part of me was actually pretty decent. His forearms – always my favorite male body part – were just the right mix of meaty and strong; the kind where you can see all the veins stand up. The amount of hair on those magical arms was masculine without looking like a gorilla. And even despite his shirt, you got an impression of the oh-so-flat abs he exhibited whenever he was able to go shirtless. Yummy! If I had to work my ass off at least the scenery was nice.

"Hi, I'm Cody," he said, as if we'd known each other for years, and put out his hand to shake mine. I thought this could be the most fun hour of working out I'd ever experienced! Thank you, Jesus.

We exchanged pleasantries then he said, "Why don't we start out with some measurements so we know what we're dealing with." He smiled as if he'd just asked me to grab lunch or something, not unveil my deepest secrets with him.

"OK," I said, a bit sheepishly. Not only had I not been honest with myself about my body and my weight, I certainly hadn't bared those personal facts and figures to anyone else, much less a young cutie like him. I gulped and wandered over to the scales he aimed me at. I held my breath, as if that was going to change anything, then watched as the digital number flashed 189. Ugh! The ugly truth.

"OK then, let's see what else you've got." And he pulled out his tape measure and started by measuring minor stuff like my neck and upper forearms before he went to the tough stuff. By that point he held the tape measure up to me, directing me to hold it to my chest for him, lest he get too personal around the girls. Chest: 42.25 inches.

I exhaled again. "Just hang in there," I whispered to my little mostly gone Mojo, "he's almost done" (I hoped) as Cody measured my waist at 40 inches. Next, the hips came in at 43, followed by my thigh at 20 and calf at 14. He did a few calculations and pronounced that my percent body fat was at 40%. (Docs like to see that number stay under 25.) Oops! Guilty!

"Ok, well that wasn't so bad, now, was it?" he smiled. I'm sure he saw people day after day at least this heavy or more, so I probably wasn't anything new on his radar. But it was surely a reality check for me. I could no longer get away with saying I wasn't "that bad." Facts were facts and the scale doesn't lie.

From there he walked me throughout various machines and free weights to see what I had as far as strength. I think I surprised him a little, for despite my numbers not being great, I'd nearly always stayed active and wasn't a complete couch potato. But by the end of our hour I was a sweaty, exhausted lump of muscles and fat who obviously needed to change my ways.

I thanked him for his time and his honesty, once I could catch my breath enough to do so. "So what do you think?" He smiled that beefcake smile again, "You want to sign up for a package of training? We've got a sale going on right now ... buy 6 get one free."

"Not right yet, Cody, but thanks. Let me get settled in a bit more and I'll see if I can't figure out which way to go soon," I said. I wiped the sweat off my hand in order to shake his, as we parted ways, then made my way to the locker room to clean up and head home. I doubted I'd ever work with him again. I still wasn't ready to work that hard.

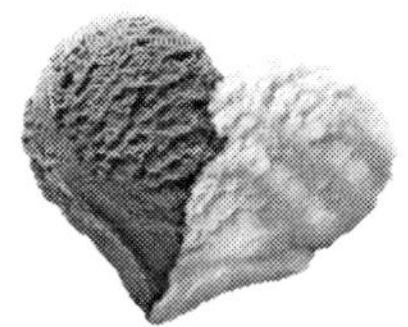

CHAPTER 12

Tryin's Lyin'

I did start going to the gym about three days a week, once I got settled into my new digs. I'd usually do 30 minutes on the bike, a few minutes on the stair stepper, maybe do a little jump-roping. Then, I'd finish it off with a little arm work. I felt like I was at least doing *something* to improve things physically; at the same time I was hoping to make some friends or at least get out of my boring house from time to time.

So I was pleased to learn that on Friday nights the gym had recreational volleyball that anyone could drop in and play. They were mostly younger than me, guys and gals who had played in high school or college some years back and still played down-and-dirty like they were competing in the Olympics or something. Big ball-hogs, frequently playing their spot and everyone else's, but for the most part it worked reasonably well. There were only a couple of old farts like me but we did fairly well considering we were a few decades older than anyone else. They didn't try to intentionally run us off the court, at any rate. There were usually more people show up than there was room for, so we had to take turns rotating in and out to give everyone a fair shot to play. The problem was biased towards those who played to win. For if you were on the winning team you got to play more. Translation: winning was everything. Sportsmanship, not so much.

At one point, I thought I'd been going long enough that I was part of the regulars, yet one night I lost my cool and couldn't go back for a few days, I was so pissed off. It went like this …

I was playing front row across the net from one of the tall, aggressive jocks who looked like if he spiked the ball in my face I'd end up in the ER or something. The ironic thing was that he was a dad to a little kid about 3 who he brought to the game every weekend. He treated that kid with such love and compassion that I guess I thought he was likely compassionate to others as well. But as we were playing I found myself in a tough spot where the server had decided I was the weak link to hit to, and put a spin on the ball just-so that I couldn't return it. The jock next to me was chomping at the bit to get his paws on the ball, I could tell, but I stayed the course and the server spun me again.

By this time, Volleyball Jock was clearly unhappy as, God forbid, we might lose the game because of my failing. (There was no prize, of course. When one game would be over, they'd just start another.) I held my place, knowing Volleyball Jock was itching to say something at the same time that the server obviously was out for blood and put his best spin on the ball yet again.

Call me a failure, but I couldn't return that man's serve to save my life! I suppose the correct things to do might have been to ask someone to switch spots with me, but I doubt it would have mattered. Odds were that, knowing I was the weakest link, he'd likely have followed me anyway, just to prove the fact that he was all that and a bag of chips. I was starting to get embarrassed when Volleyball Jock finally said to me, "Just move," as he took over my spot, essentially dismissing me from any further play. The hunger in his eyes quite evident that he was only concerned for the win!

I lost it. I don't even remember the exact words I said, but I do remember poking him with my index finger in the chest, over and over, scolding him for being an ass. Something like, "Take your fucking ball and stuff it!" I hoped that I made him feel as though his mom was giving him a tongue lashing in public. If he hadn't been so darn tall I might have even been able to grab him by the ear and pull his face down to my level and gotten his attention that way! I suspect it took him off guard at least. I finally stopped pounding my finger in his skin and turned and left the court, heading for the hot tub.

I'd gone there to have fun with some folks, I fumed. No pressure. Just relaxing fun with a little exercise thrown in. Why did some people have to make everything such a big deal? It's no wonder some folks would rather stay home than even try to get in shape, if they were only going to be belittled at the damned gym. I was building a full head of steam.

Thank God for the Jacuzzi. I loved that Jacuzzi. The jets were perfect, it was big enough to hold abut eight people, and they maintained it pretty well, usually. I especially loved it when no one was there but me and I'd close my eyes and float away with the bubbles, my mind and body going floaty-floaty in the jets that were always trying their darnedest (or so it seemed) to pull my bathing suit off with their turbulence. That night I needed this more than anything.

The hot tub was also where friendships were born and, in fact, that's where I met my great friend, Mary Ann.

She was 72 years old and had been widowed and retired several years earlier. She was about 5 feet, 4 inches tall and 100 pounds dripping wet. Her body was rock hard without an ounce of fat to be found. She had very short hair that had probably once been a sort of sandy color but now was being blended into grey with auburn streaks sneaking in among her waves. Her alabaster skin showed that she'd never been a sun worshipper and being Irish, her paleness glowed through. And when she walked around that gym, people noticed. She seemed to glide, rather than walk. Kind of like a runway model, she held her body in a manner that said, "I know who I am."

She was intensely independent, lived alone with just her dog (her only son far off in Oregon), and was a gym rat like no other. Come to find out she'd been a marathon runner most of her adult life and it showed. There were few women in that gym on any given day of the week who could hold a candle to Mary Ann. And she was proud of that fact, although she'd never admit to it. She didn't work out to be pretty. She didn't care what anyone thought of her routines or how much weight she could lift or how many minutes she could pump the rowing machine. She simply did it because she loved the way her body felt when she was in shape.

Her routine put me to shame. On Tuesdays, Thursdays, and Saturday mornings she went to yoga class. After that she would go home and have lunch. (She lived only a few blocks away.) Then she'd come back those same afternoons to swim or water-walk for an hour. On Mondays, Wednesdays, and

 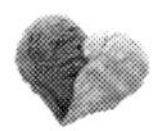

Fridays she did weights and cardio on her own, moving from the arm cycle to free weights, to the rowing machine and more. She had an established routine. To finish out the week, on Sunday she would swim or water walk for yet another hour. No days off. No scoffing off. Yet, while she was dead serious about her fitness, that didn't preclude her from laughing and playing and joking around with everyone. Her laugh echoed when she'd start giggling at something and would pull others in to do the same. In the vastness of the pool area, her giggles echoed off the damp ceramic walls, the bouncing only further elongating the sounds into something curiously unhuman-like.

The gym was her community. That's where her friends were. It wasn't work for her. Rather, it was what she lived for. Little did she know at that time just how valuable all those years of fitness would turn out to be. A few years later she suffered (and recovered from) a stroke and moved to Oregon to be near her son, leaving a huge hole in my heart. I missed her like crazy.

But, getting back to my story, just as with me, the best parts for her at the gym were the hot tub and the steam room.

I still remember our chats in the tub and how we really got a connection over a discussion about what type of footwear to have on while pool walking. Since the pool surface was rough to keep from being slippery, it also had a tendency to scratch the heck out of your feet. It became quite our experiment and we ended up agreeing that an old pair of clean tennies was the way to go.

It took a while before Mary Ann and I got close, though. I must have asked her to go out to lunch with me four or five times and she always declined. I even invited her to my family's Thanksgiving, knowing she would otherwise spend it alone, but nope. Nothing doing.

What I figured out over time was that she needed to say no to something at least four times and then she'd do it. I guess she wanted to know I was serious about whatever I was proposing. But despite that and no matter our age difference, we became each other's "go to" person and watching the effort she put into caring for her body, I started to push myself a bit more as well. Just not too much at first.

***

November 2008

"I'm getting married, Mom!" My daughter, Shaun, age 25, was a year away from graduating from medical school in Kansas City. She'd called to tell me the news and could hardly contain herself. She and her fiancé, Bill, had been together for several years and I had expected they would tie the knot sometime. Looked like the time had come.

"Do you have a date in mind?" I queried, feeling a new excitement growing that would keep us all busy for a while.

"Well, we thought we'd elope and save you and Dad a bunch of money!" She was teasing, but kept playing it up a bit. "That work for you?" I could tell Bill was trying to tickle her at the same time, as she started giggling like a school girl while still trying to talk.

"Oh, no you don't! We're gonna have a wedding," I replied. "I've only got one daughter and by God I'm going to get one wedding! So, now that that's settled, do you have a date in mind?"

She giggled again and I could sense the happiness between them. It was a good fit. I couldn't have been luckier with my soon-to-be new son-in-law!

"Well, with graduation and my internship starting right after that, the only time we really have would be the end of May. Like Memorial Day weekend. Would that work? That leaves us about eight months to plan as well."

"Consider it on the calendar!" I said.

I was so happy for the news, but at the same time I suddenly had this image in my head of all those wedding pictures that were going to be taken, which of course would last for blooming-ever, AND my ex-husband who would be there as well. Well, okay, it wasn't a bad thing that he was going to be there. We got along well enough. We just didn't seek each other out any more … unless the subject was our daughter.

But somehow my little Mojo voice instantly felt vulnerable. My ex had been dating someone for quite a while – in fact he ended up marrying her after Shaun's wedding was behind us. And I, was once again ... er ... single.

Bottom line: For this wedding, I wanted to look hot!

Reality check: I was not looking anywhere near hot!

Analysis: I had 8 months to get my butt in gear and really make some changes, if I meant it.

And, oh, boy, did I mean it! I called Cody the next day to set up a training schedule.

***

My next workout with Cody was on November 12, 2008. It had been seven months since our first encounter and I sadly admitted that I hadn't produced any improvements working out on my own, not even with all the extra summer activities like biking and hiking I'd added to my three-day-a-week gym workouts. Of course those great summer calorie-burning activities were probably cancelled out by the extra summer BBQ'S and cookouts I'd attended with the accompanying chips, hot dogs, cakes and pies I had managed to over-eat. And of course with the holiday season not far off, there was plenty of danger to come.

I explained to Cody that I had eight months to get ready for this wedding and that I was 100 percent committed to the work. In fact, I had never been so intent on a goal as I was that one. I had learned a great lesson about intention and commitment a long time ago from a dear friend named Joe, who was listening to me doing what I thought was my best whining about why no diet I ever tried had worked. We were sitting in a busy coffee shop, and he'd been pretty quiet for a while as I was ranting on. At last, he turned to me and said, "MJ, I want you to do something for me, OK?" He had one of those looks on his face that told me he was serious but also that he'd just as likely pull a rabbit out of his hat any minute. He was a bit my senior, had been around the world a time or two with various jobs he'd held, and had raised a family, so I figured he'd likely have some experiences that could be helpful.

Tentatively, I said, "OK ... I think." Wondering just what I'd walked into this time.

He pointed to my coffee cup and said, "Try to pick up that cup."

I looked at him, confused. "I don't get it," I replied.

He kept his poker face on and asked again, "Just try to pick up your cup."

I gave him a stupid look, still waiting for the rabbit to jump out of the cup. But at last, I slowly lifted up the cup a good 12 inches off the table. Holding it there, feeling ridiculous.

He shook his head, grinning and said, "I didn't ask you to PICK up the cup ... I only asked you to TRY to pick up the cup." I looked even more confused and set my cup down again.

He continued, "This is DO," he said, and he picked up the cup. He held it there for a long moment, then set it back down. "This is DON'T DO," and he took his hand away from the cup. Again, pausing. Hoping it was getting through to me, I guess. "And this," he held his hand over the cup, acting as though he was straining to pick it up but as if it were glued to the table, and it wouldn't budge. "*This* is tryin'." He held the pose for another few seconds, then set it down, grinning.

"Tryin's lyin', Sweetheart."

"I still don't get it," I was really confused by then.

Joe chuckled. "You remember in *Star Wars* when Luke Skywalker went to his Jedi training with Yoda out in the boonies? It's the same theory. 'There is no TRY. Only Do or Don't Do,' he would growl at Luke, who was only putting out half-assed effort (*trying*) under Yoda's tutelage. Luke had every excuse in the book why his aim was off or why he couldn't see with his helmet shield down, necessitating him to use his abilities through pure focus and not just his five senses. Once he finally quit whining and ran out of excuses and accepted nothing less than success was he able to sail through his testing and walk out the other side a Jedi."

I was remembering that scene vividly and was finally making some sense of what he'd been demonstrating. He had gone on, "If your intention is not a hundred percent to do something, then don't even start. Even with an intention of 99 percent, that one percent that's not on board can sabotage whatever you're doing before you even get started."

I had been down that road plenty of times before …

Being the writer I am, words are like power tools to me. So, with all that combined, I was determined that there would be no Tryin' for me, only Doin'. After that, I became very conscious of using the word "try" in any of my conversations with anyone about anything and was amazed how obvious it was which people were *doing* and which were just *trying*; whether at work or weight loss or anything.

If you want to prove it to yourself, just ask some folks over for a get together that involves helping with some big project (painting or something), then sit back and see which ones say they'll try to be there and those who say they will be there. By the time it's over, I bet very few of the Tryers ever make it. Cuz they weren't committed to it to start with. And they let their subconscious minds (that never really wanted to go to begin with) call the shots despite their conscious mind believing it really ran the show and had every intention of going. Beware that subconscious mind and its power.

Word to the wise: If you're going to take on some kind of challenge – especially one as complex as weight loss – be sure your intention is one hundred percent or simply don't waste your time faking it. Your time is worth more than that. And why be miserable if you already know your outcome will be less than you hope for to begin with? 'Nuf said.

So I signed up for twice a week workouts with Cody and I planned to work out a total of six days per week over the lunch hour, logging all my workouts and weight info in a journal. I promptly went out and bought a cool vibrant-pink journal with a bunch of cartoon animals on it, in which I recorded all the info from my first session with Cody from way back in April. I cringed seeing those terrible numbers but thought to myself that I'd be making a dent in that real soon. And that one day I'd look back at this journal for posterity's sake (which actually turned out to be the case, or you wouldn't be reading this book right now!) I wrote the headline: Begin the Journey!

Next I dug out a calendar just to keep in the bathroom to document my weight every day, knowing I could transfer that info to the journal when it was convenient.

As usual, I would weigh every morning after my morning trip to the bathroom, which would either set a positive tone for the day if the number that greeted me was in my favor, or else a determination renewed for the day's planned activities if it didn't.

I put myself together a new gym bag. Filled it with a new set of weight lifting gloves, towel, magazine, and water bottle. Yep, I was as ready as I was going to get.

"Let's get this show rolling," I said, eager to see just how much I could lose by getting serious.

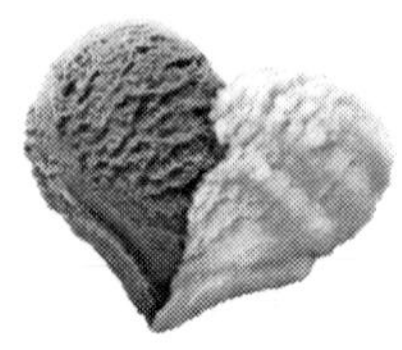

CHAPTER 13

Working Hard But...

My work began on November 6, 2008. Nearly every day I'd head to the gym over the lunch hour and dive into my program. Here's what my journal says I did throughout the month of November, and boy – will you be surprised to see what happened. So no sneaking now – don't jump ahead to see how much weight I lost. Rather, check out how hard I worked and what a gym rat I became on this mission of mine. I think you'll be surprised. I know I was. Although it wasn't what I anticipated, exactly.

Nov. 6 Gym workout 45 minutes plus a few free weights.
Nov. 8 Stationary bike 45 minutes plus a few free weights.
Nov. 10 Workout with Cody. Machines. Abs.
Nov. 12 Workout with Cody. Cardio and machines.
Nov. 13 Cardio 45 minutes. Bike. Stepper. Row.
Nov. 14 100 steps on stepper plus free weights.
Nov.16 Rode real bike 32 miles in wind! 2 hours and 40 minutes! Nice day!
Nov. 17 Mix it up workout with Cody.
Nov. 18 Real bike ride in park 45 minutes. Ten miles.

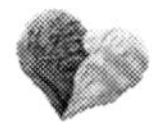

Nov. 19 Workout with Cody abs.
Nov. 20 Cardio 1 hour on various machines.
Nov. 21 Workout with Cody - machines.
Nov. 22 Bike ride for 22 miles!
Nov. 23 Bike ride 15 miles – crashed and had to walk back! Ouch.
Nov. 25 Cardio 45 minutes plus 5 minutes on the hated climbing machine.
Nov. 26 Workout with Cody weights plus extra 20 minutes cardio.
Nov. 27 Swim 20 minutes.
Nov. 28 Workout with Cody mix it up cardio plus machines.
Nov. 30 Swim 25.

November raced by as I kept my eye on the goal. The wedding date was set for June 6. I had 7 months to whip this body into shape.

I was committed to this program and was delighted to see my improvements in terms of my strength and stamina right away. My first days of pushing myself I increased my ho-hum workout (pre-Cody) efforts of maybe 20 minutes cardio, to 30 and then not long after, 45. I'd also gone from just walking briskly on the treadmill, with a mild incline to starting to jog – which I hated. My knees had taken a hammering throughout my lifetime, from all those athletic activities of youth. Then, add years of riding jumping horses, which put intense pressure on my knees with every stride, I'd beaten them up royally and they didn't hesitate in reminding me often. So I did what I could cardio-wise, avoiding jogging as much as possible, but throwing it in here and there just to see how my stamina was doing.

Despite all this, my weight hadn't seemed to move much, which left me a bit nervous. Cody had told me to stay away from the every-day weighing I liked to do and instead he only wanted me to weigh once per month. His philosophy was in part that some of the changes I would undergo would be building more muscle, which was great. But, that also came with some extra pounds in the beginning and he didn't want me to get discouraged. And so, despite almost going through withdrawals without my scale, I didn't dare step on it except for once per month.

By the end of the first month I couldn't wait to hit that scale and maybe even take some measurements to grab on to any little detail that would give me evidence that all this hard work was working!

I raced into the gym on December 1, peeled off my jacket and heavy outside clothing. Pulled on my workout shorts and top as fast as I could move. Grabbed my tennis shoes, water bottle, and workout gloves and headed for the scale in the trainer's office. I decided to weigh myself before Cody arrived so that I could tease him when he got there, maybe having him guess just how much I'd lost. I was hoping for maybe five pounds at least.

I jumped on the scale and closed my eyes and held my breath as the digital numbers calibrated and then finally landed on a steady number.

I excitedly opened my eyes and instantly crashed with disappointment. 188 pounds!

 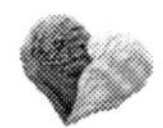

ONE POUND?! That couldn't possibly be! I had worked my ass off five days per week for four weeks in a row to lose one measly pound? I could have lost one pound by just not drinking for a day! What the hell?

My mind raced back over the month's activities, wondering where I had gone wrong. That just couldn't be right.

I did admit that my original intention had been to workout six times per week and as I looked back over my journal (which I always brought to show Cody or to keep track of anything new we were working on), I counted up the November workouts and realized it only added up to five workouts per week. OK, so there was that. While it wasn't the complete answer, it definitely didn't help the situation. I wondered how I'd let that happen, though ... especially since I felt like I lived there every single day for the whole bloody month!

Of course, there was Thanksgiving ... it had only been several days before and I remembered pigging out on absolutely everything: turkey, dressing, mashed potatoes, gravy, rolls, sweet potato casserole, pumpkin and cherry pie, dump cake (my contribution...my favorite high-sugar, holiday binge food!) And don't forget the appetizers on the front end of the meal. My sister's famous clam dip, the sausage and crackers. The chips and dips. But certainly I'd worn that off by now, hadn't I?

I was more than a little upset. I was damned angry. And had I found out this information at home I'd likely have thrown quite a fit. Fortunately for my dog, who would have had to endure my temper tantrum, I got most of it out in the workout, but not before Cody arrived and saw how upset I was.

"It's OK, it's OK," he said, trying to calm me down. "It's only the first month. Your body is going through a lot of changes. It's building up a lot of muscle as I warned you about."

I *did* remember his earlier lecture about that. But surely, my body could have let go of just a little more!? While my goal was still firmly in place, with only seven months now to reach it, I could feel a little waver in the old commitment department. The little Miss Mojo voice I'd felt so good about all month was downright sad and suddenly felt weak at the same time.

"How are you doing with the food," Cody asked, gently. Still trying to make light of the situation.

I could barely hear him through my anger. "What?"

"I asked how you're doing with the food?" He picked up his clipboard and pen as we were about to head out to start the day's workout.

"Doing *what* with the food?" My lips were moving as I answered but my brain wasn't registering. He may as well have been speaking Russian to me. I nodded my head, only halfway present and said, "Fine, fine. I'm eating healthy. Oatmeal for breakfast. You know ... that kind of thing." I honestly didn't hear another word he said for the rest of our session.

An hour later, after working me out for all that it was worth, I headed to the locker room, dressed in a flash to get out of there, and went home to cry half the night on my couch, curled up with my dog and a half a gallon of Blue Bunny ice cream. Of course by morning I was like the guilty drunk with a hangover. Guilt and remorse. Guilt and remorse. Yet feeling justified all the same.

***

 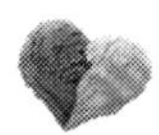

If November had been disappointing, December was a disaster. Definitely not the best month to expect great success in terms of weight loss, even for those with the best of intentions. While I had kept up with the workouts, even closer to six days a week this time, I had certainly done nothing to steer clear of all the food that was around every corner.

Christmas cookies were everywhere! Of course there was fudge galore. (A little bit of heaven, if you ask me.) Then there were the mini loaves of banana, cranberry, and chocolate chip/pumpkin bread that my friend Nancy gave out to everyone on her gift list each year. (Yum!) I think I attended at least three Christmas parties (not including Christmas day itself), where I gorged on fancy mixed nuts, chocolate mint candies, and chocolate truffles that melted in my mouth in a heart beat. The chocolate/peppermint bark was to die for.

Oh yeah, did I say I had a friend's wedding to attend as well, where on top of all the usual holiday fare there was wedding cake too?

All in all, it was an especially happy holiday season for me as I had been invited to spend several days with my daughter, her fiancé Bill, and Bill's young son, Dawson, in Kansas City. With her crazy life as a medical student occupying her life full-time and then some, it was rare for me to get to spend more than a handful of days with her each year, so I was thrilled for the visit. And to add to the fun we even made our own Christmas cookies and decorated them. God, I love frosted Christmas cookies! My sugar addiction was in full gear. I knew I was stuffing myself but the holidays would be over soon and I could get back to my normal eating/working out schedule soon. No problem.

Oh yeah, on top of everything else, throw my birthday in there, (Christmas Eve), and Christmas Day family feast, PLUS New Year's Eve festivities … and guess what?

My weight clocked in for December at 196 pounds!

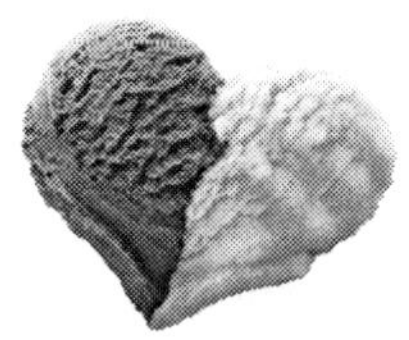

CHAPTER 14

You Can't Outrun The Fork — It's Got Two More Legs Than You!

One day, not soon after the holidays, I must have been brooding about the number on the scales again when one of the trainers named Bernie struck up a conversation with me. Bernie had retired from his professional career several years back and then, sometime after that he'd become a personal trainer for his groupies who adored him. He was from Bahstun (that's Boston with a very thick accent) and was quite the card. He must have stood over six feet tall, was in great shape, still had a head of thick, gray hair, a perky grey mustache, and wore glasses from time to time when reading. Did I mention he was fit, fit, fit? Yet another one of those guys who made even a t-shirt look hot, hot, hot as it clung to his well-formed pectoral muscles as well as his abs. Only years of work could make a body look like that. Yet he had no pretentiousness about him whatsoever.

And boy, did he know how to flirt! I don't think he cared which women he flirted with, they were all lovely to him. His devilish grin always left you wondering if he was teasing or not. But we all knew it was all just play.

"So, how's it going there, Gorgeous?" he inquired of me as I was waiting for Cody to show up. Bernie gave me a look that was definitely a "once over" type of glance. As if he could tell whether Cody was a good trainer or not depending on what he saw of my body in a quick glance.

"Oh, Bernie. I'm so frustrated," I muttered, having just weighed myself yet again with still no success. "I've been working out like a crazy person for four months – you've seen me – and while Cody assures me that I'm doing great, and I'm definitely getting stronger, I'm just not losing any weight. It's very disappointing."

I stretched my legs to get ready for the workout, bending from the waist and laying my palms flat on the floor. At least one thing I was still pretty good at was flexibility.

"And what about the food?" he questioned.

I fell back on my standard line. "Yeah, I'm eating pretty healthy. Oatmeal for breakfast, yogurt, fruit, some meat. Weight Watchers meals." Long pause. "And I admit to eating way too much sugar." I was embarrassed for my confession but I couldn't lie to Bernie. At least not like I'd been lying to myself for the last four months. I knew if I would only eliminate the junk food from my diet, it would make a big difference. It sounded so easy but the addiction was so powerful. And junk food was the mainstay of my diet!

And of course filling my body with food seemed to always make me feel better – for a while. That hole in my life, where there was no man to share it with, among other things, seemed not to be so deep whenever I was stuffing food into it.

"I hate to tell you this, Kiddo, but in case Cody hasn't explained this clearly, weight loss is about 80 percent food and

 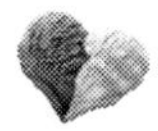

20 percent exercise. And unless you've got that 80 percent working for you rather than against you, you'll never win the battle with the scales." I stood up from my stretching position, face red from being upside down, but also from pure embarrassment at my denial.

Bernie continued, "No one can work out enough each day to burn all those extra calories. Unless you're an Olympic athlete who works out five to six hours a day and who eats three or four thousand calories per day during intensive training, just to maintain their weight. I assume you're not one of those people?"

I shook my head. "Well, the bottom line is this," he went on. "You can't outrun the fork. Or the spoon or the straw or whatever vehicle you're using to inhale your food. Cuz, honey – it's got two more legs than you!"

About that time Cody arrived and Bernie gave him one of his "I told you so" looks. "Haven't you been teaching her about the food? What's wrong with you, Mr. Body Builder?"

Cody didn't quite know what to say, but offered, "I tried. She said she was doing OK with that. I can't force her." And he was right.

"It's not his fault," I interrupted. "He has asked me several times what I was doing about what I'm eating and I just wasn't ready to go there yet, I guess. But now I'm getting desperate. I'm running out of time. And I don't know what to do." I started to tear up. The many weeks of hard work with almost no visible results had just about maxed me out. And the guys knew they had pushed me to the edge.

"OK, OK," Bernie said. "You look like you need a hug," and he put his arms around me in a big bear hug and about squeezed the stuffing right out of me.

When he finally let me go, Cody stepped in to give me a hug as well. Since it was the closest thing to male physical contact that I'd had for a good, long while, I ate it up!

"Alright then. I know Cody's your trainer but obviously you could use another cheerleader in your corner. Am I right?" He smiled his devilish smile again, putting his hands on my shoulders and pulling my slumping body up to attention. "Your homework is to journal your food from every day forward. I mean everything that goes in your mouth – healthy or unhealthy. And I want exact measurements. If you eat grapes, either write down how many individually or how many cups. If you eat a bacon cheeseburger, you write down all the individual items that goes in that burger – all the cheese, the bacon, ketchup, the bun – all of it.

"Next, you get yourself an education about calories and portions. Start looking up how many calories are in the foods you eat every day. You know how to read labels, I assume? Every package of anything in the store now has nutritional information on it, so you don't even have much investigating to do."

I tried to look thankful as Bernie laid out the plan, but my inner good and evil voices had already begun to sneak into the back of my mind. I felt like I had my little devil on one shoulder saying, "You don't want to do that, do you? Sure sounds like a lot of work to me. What fun is that?"

And on my other shoulder, my Miss Mojo saying, "This is awesome! Finally an answer to help you hit that goal that you really, really know you want to reach." I tried not to let my inner avatars doing battle show through in my expression as I concentrated while Bernie nailed down every detail as to what he expected.

 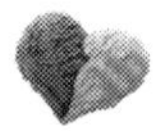

"Sure, you've got to put a little work in to start with, but once you familiarize yourself with the information it will come easily. You already keep a workout journal, don't you?" I nodded, not too sure what I was getting myself into. "Well, this is just another part of the equation that you've already been keeping records for. And it's the piece that should get you off dead center." Bernie laughed. "Oh come on, you look like somebody died. You should be looking like you just won the lottery!"

"Thanks, guys. I really appreciate all your help." I gave them my best fake smile and figured it was time to get to work with Cody when he chimed in, "Hey Bernie. Is that BodyBugg promo still going on? Maybe that would be a good idea for her."

I looked back and forth from one of them to the other, not having a clue what they were talking about. "What's that?" I asked. Curious but cautious. God knows what they were getting me into. I was still adjusting to the idea of having to count calories, for God's sake!

"Cody, for once your brain is thinking!" He turned to me and said, "You've seen the *Biggest Loser* show on TV, right?"

"Sure," I replied. "I watch it." I was becoming mildly interested.

"Well, have you seen the things they wear on their upper arms? It's like a stretchy black strap attached to some little tech tool. I don't know how it works but they somehow track a lot of data with it." Bernie looked to Cody for more depth of explanation since computer stuff was not his forte.

Cody took over, "It works with your computer both downloading your data regarding calories burned with your input regarding what you're eating. I think it also tracks proteins, carbs, and fats too. *The Biggest Loser* is apparently having great luck with them and right now we've got a promo going that if you buy a ten training-session package, you get a free Body-Bugg. They usually run about $200 otherwise."

"This could be your ticket, Kiddo," Bernie's positive energy was starting to flow over to me. I looked back and forth from one to the other and asked, "Where do I get mine?"

***

The first thing I finally learned to accept is that there is no magic secret to losing weight. In its simplest terms, it's all about calories-in versus calories-out. I like to think of it like my check book: If I have $1,500 in my check book and then I write a check for $1,500, I can't make any further purchases until I have more money in the check book. How does that translate to calories? If I want to limit myself to eating say 1,500 calories today, then once I've consumed 1,500, my bank is empty and there are no more calories available for me today. At least not until the next day when the bank gets a new daily, automatic deposit to work with and I start again. It's truly that simple. And I wasted so many months fighting that fact.

Most of us don't want to write down what we eat, not so much because it's tedious, or a bit time-consuming, but because it's a visual reminder of many not-so-great choices we've made. When you see that 600 calories of ice cream for breakfast in your log book it's just damned embarrassing! It's bad enough when I see it, much less if I have to show it to my trainer!

 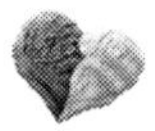

I decided that if I invested a little bit of time to learn all the specifics and ins-and-outs of calories and portions, it would be worth it. Besides, the weight wasn't going to fall off all by itself. If that were the case, everyone would be thin. But if my goal was to lose the weight yet still be able to eat anything that I wanted (which it still was, and always would be) then I needed to understand the roadmap on how to get there. I knew that for me I could commit to focusing on one thing: calories. I knew I would still eat things that were bad for me, but at least the decisions would be mine and I would know what they added up to.

I'm not super techie, so I was a little bit intimidated by the BodyBugg at first but I'd been watching the folks on the Biggest Loser use theirs and it didn't look too horrible. I signed up for the online part, which is where I would input what I ate each day. Then, the tracker itself would calculate my calories burned based upon my body temperature, sweat, and who knows what scientific algorithms they were working with. It wasn't waterproof (although many of today's trackers are) so I had to manually enter info regarding my time water walking or swimming.

It proved to be pretty easy to use, actually, and I liked the instant feedback I got at the end of each day telling me my calorie burn, and if I was above or below where I wanted to be. As for tracking the food, even that was pretty easy. For example, I had Quaker Instant Oatmeal for breakfast every day. Once I entered the nutritional info for that product, all I had to say the next morning was yes – I had the same thing for breakfast today and it automatically filled in the info for me. It also told me how many grams of carbs, proteins, and fats I'd eaten. Which was more info than I really wanted to keep track of but Bernie and Cody were big on that.

I rearranged my entire workout log to reflect not only the exercise that I'd been doing, but now all the BodyBugg info as well. My start date was March 21 and my weight was still stuck at 191#.

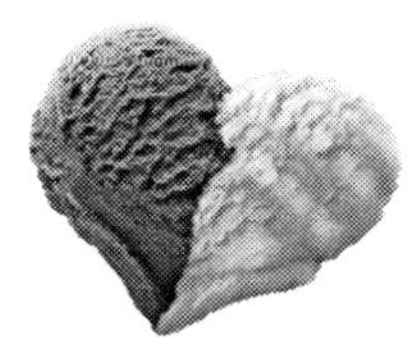

CHAPTER 15

It All Adds Up...

I spent a couple of hours one afternoon learning the calorie counts and portions for several food items, most of which were the foods I normally ate, or else foods I was simply curious about. Some really surprised me. Especially what some companies counted as a serving! (Note: T = tablespoon)

Dorito's Nacho Cheese Chips (11 chips) .... 240 calories
(Who eats just 11 chips?!)

Guacamole (2T) 40
(Surely I don't eat more than that!)

Wendy's cheeseburger 270

Wendy's medium fries 420

Subway 6-inch tuna sandwich.................. 530

Subway six-inch meatball sandwich 580

Subway six-inch sweet onion chicken teriyaki.................................. 370

Little Caesar's lunch combo, 1 slice 360
They come four slices per box. Who eats just one? Come on, admit it. Most people would easily have two and many would eat all four! You do the math!)

Taco Bell Tacos 170
(If I order these I usually get three, which equals 510)

Taco Bell Chicken quesadilla 510

Taco Bell taco salad . . . . 770!
(That greasy shell will get you every time! There are 200 or more calories just in the shell.)

Peanut Butter and Jelly Sandwich 330
(Varies depending on type of bread as well as jelly.)

Grilled cheese sandwich . . . . 350 - 600
(Depending on how much cheese, what kind of bread, and how much butter is used)

Mac and cheese (1 cup) 320

Salmon (4 ounces - grilled) 200

Chicken (4 ounces - grilled) 200

Steak (4 ounces - grilled) 230

Chocolate glazed cake donut 400

Hostess cupcake (one) 160
(Of course in my mind, a serving is one container worth, which, of course is two cupcakes!), therefore 320 calories. (Maybe I'll eat only 1? ... Not likely!)

Ben and Jerry's Cherry Garcia Ice Cream, 1 pint. . . . . 960!!!
(Their serving size is 1/2 cup and there are 4 servings per pint. My serving size equals the whole thing! Honestly, what were they thinking?)

Large movie theatre popcorn tub without butter 1,000
(By adding butter this number can go up by the hundreds.)

Dairy Queen's Oreo Cookies Blizzard (medium) 790

Snickers candy bar (regular size) 250

Snickers candy bar (king size). 440

Apple 100

Banana. 100

Red grapes (1 cup). 100

Orange juice (1 cup) 100

Light yogurt 80

Regular yogurt 200

Egg 55

Frosted flakes cereal (1 cup) 147
(Odds are you eat closer to 2 cups.)

English muffin 150

Strawberry jam (2 T)............................35

Butter (1 T)..................................100

Mayonnaise (1T)...............................60

Ranch salad dressing (1T)..................... 43

Sour cream (1T)...............................20

Bacon (1 slice)...............................40

Mixed nuts (1/4 cup).........................170
(I don't know about you, but I'd eat at least
3 times that! Yum!)

Whole Milk (1 cup)...........................150

2% Milk (1 cup)..............................130

1% Milk (1 cup)..............................113

Skim Milk (1 cup)............................ 80

Soda regular (1 can).........................140

Wine (white or red - small glass)............200

Beer (12 ounce bottle).......................120

Tequila (shot)...............................100

Coffee (black).................................0

Tea (non-sweetened)............................0

I was astounded at this information – especially as it pertained to exactly what a portion was, like with the Ben

 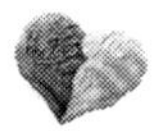

and Jerry's confusion! I mean, come on – who on Earth eats one half a cup of ice cream as a serving? Certainly not those people who are sugar addicts like me!

Then there were other deceiving things, like the taco salad at Taco Bell. I think I'll eat a healthy salad at lunch today. That will be good for me. Never suspecting that I'd eat up 770 of my day's calories in no time! It's crazy, but that taco shell alone is loaded with calories. I learned that I could actually eat the salad and leave the shell, still enjoying a salad but shaving off those extra 200 calories – although I admit, that's the best part! However, as I made my choice between 200 calories from a taco shell versus using that 200 calories for something like an ounce of fudge, and still come out using 80 less than had I eaten the damned edible bowl, the fudge was gonna win every time.

I also tuned in to serving sizes a little more with the Weight Watchers, Lean Cuisine, and Healthy Choice frozen, light meals I ate. It hit me loud and clear that what they were imagining to be a portion size in those little plastic containers was certainly not the amount of food I would normally be scooping onto my plate for myself. I actually kept a few of those little plastic trays that the meals come in to use as a guide when serving myself at home. For example, if I made spaghetti for dinner, I would measure out my serving in the Weight Watcher's container and by the way – I had to be able to cover the dish with Saran Wrap or aluminum foil to make it level, otherwise it would be too easy to just keep piling it higher and higher if I wasn't careful!

Then, there were the seemingly little things that added up really quickly like 2 tablespoons of butter registering in at 200 calories, or the same amount of mayonnaise at 120. Those things never seemed like much when I was buttering my bread but, again, if I'm spending 200 calories from my imaginary check book, I'd rather have chocolate than butter! The butter was just too "“expensive” for me!

And when it came to eating out, the smartest thing in terms of portion control for me was to have the waiter divide my serving into two; putting one half on my dinner plate and one half in a to-go box before the meal even landed at my table. Yet one more way to stay on track.

Food is so ingrained in our culture as either a reward for things well done, or as a Band-aid when things go wrong. You have a bad day at work? Eat something! Just got a raise? Celebrate – eat something! Mom worked hard all day preparing a feast? Don't make her feel like she didn't work hard enough. Eat up! And of course, have seconds!

Honestly, one of our biggest problems as an overweight nation is that most people don't have a clue as to what a reasonable portion size even looks like. Making it worse, every fast-food company keeps super-sizing each and every meal. It is so easy to blindly say yes to that faceless voice that always asks, “Would you like to super-size that?” We always think that bigger must be better.

Is it any wonder we have trouble losing weight?

One thing caught my eye lately as I was standing in the grocery check-out line. Suddenly all the candy bars that are put there intentionally to catch your eye and get you to drooling have jumped to KING SIZE! What? It wasn't tempting enough to wave a 250-calorie Snickers right in front of me, they had to upsize that as well to King Size with 440 calories!

And how many folks really notice, as their 4 year old begs Mommy for a candy bar and threatens a tantrum at the grocery store if he doesn't get it?

Here's another example: Guess how many calories are in a 32-ounce Super Big Gulp regular Coke? 621! And that's not the biggest size out there any more!

Just to give myself another glimpse as to what all this information could teach me on my journey, I put together some examples of how some of these foods added up in what I considered a normal day's calorie intake ...

Breakfast:
Orange juice (1 cup) 100
Bacon (2 slices) 80
Eggs (2) 110
English muffin 150
Jam (2 T) 35
Butter (2 T) 200

TOTAL 675

Lunch:
Subway 6 inch meatball sandwich 580
Bag of chips 240
Cookies (2) 420
Coke (1 can) 120

TOTAL 1,360

Dinner:
Mac and cheese (1 cup) 320

Peanut butter and jelly sandwich 330

TOTAL 650

After dinner:
Movie theatre popcorn
(1/2 of large tub) 500
(Sharing the other half with someone – hopefully!)

TOTAL FOR THE DAY . . . . 3,185!!!!

My daily calorie allowance when in losing mode: About 1,400! No surprise I kept gaining weight so easily when I study these numbers!

Does this seem extreme? It's not! It's simply not that hard to just keep eating all day long. Looking back over my journal I hate to admit that I hit the 3,000 calorie number a few times, usually over a holiday or some other event. Or, honestly, when I simply fell off the wagon.

So, what was a normal calorie requirement for one day, I wondered? Since we are all different, I learned that there is a pretty wide range of answers to that question, factoring in gender differences, height, activity level, and age. In other words, if you're sedentary, your requirements will obviously be much lower than someone who pushes a lawn mower all day. It was important that I figure out how many calories my body burned on an average day so that I could then figure out an ideal number of calories I should limit myself to each day.

So, back to the BodyBugg I went. Each day I tracked calories-in as well as calories burned. After a few days I started to see that my body was burning around 2,500 to 3,000 each day, and that was counting all my working out. So, if I aimed for about 1,700 to 2,000 calories as my calories-in limit each day, that would leave me a net loss of 500 to 1,300 calories-out.

Sure sounded easy on paper!

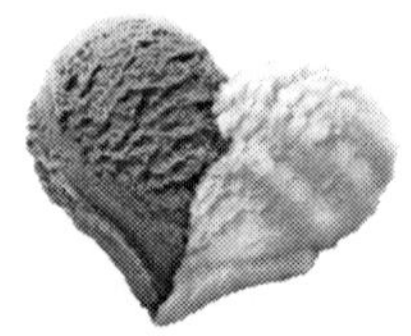

CHAPTER 16

The Race To The Wire

Now, with all my new knowledge in place, it was time to really get serious about tracking my food. Of course fessing up to what I was really eating was the most humbling step of all and I went over my info with Cody once a week as part of our training time. And because I was being honest about what I ate, I obviously didn't eat quite as much junk food as usual because I didn't want another lecture from him. So I balanced my good side with my bad side.

As such, a typical day of eating for me would be:

Breakfast: Instant Oatmeal - 2 packs: 300 calories
Snack: 2 Tablespoons of peanut butter: 200 calories
Lunch: Weight Watcher's meal: 350 calories
Snack: Candy bar: 250 calories
Dinner: Grilled chicken and vegetables: 400 calories
Snack: Light popcorn: 150 calories
Total: 1650
Total calories burned all day per bodybugg: 2650
Therefore total deficit: 1000 calories burned away.

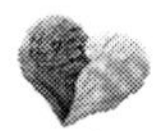

Since it takes approximately 3,500 calories to equal one pound of fat, in 3-1/2 days of similar workout-to-food ratio, I should be able to drop one pound.

A couple other days' intakes might be:
Breakfast: Light yogurt - 80 with
Red grapes (2 cups) - 200
Lunch: Weight Watcher meal - 350
Snack: Cookies, 2 large - 500
Dinner: Microwave popcorn - 250
Snack: Apple - 100

Total: 1,480

Or, another day it might look like this:

Breakfast: 2 Donuts - 800
Lunch: 2 cups Cantaloupe -120
Snack: Protein bar - 250
Dinner: Weight Watcher's Meal - 180

Total: 1,350

BY THE WAY - I NEVER DRINK MY CALORIES!

Water, coffee, or unsweetened ice tea are your stand-bys. If you must drink your calories, then you'll have to deduct something else to make up for it.

I stuck like glue to the plan and believe it or not, in ten days I lost 5 pounds! I still ate pizza or candy or ice cream, but it all had to fit into my daily calorie allowance. Oh yeah – and I ate at least one healthy thing per day.

Holy Moly! After how many months of frustrating results, it suddenly became perfectly clear to me: I can't outrun the fork! Bernie was right ... it's all about the food!

Don't get me wrong – all the workouts I'd spent hours doing at the gym over all those months were not in vain. My stamina and strength had made some huge leaps. Without listing my full routines again, suffice it to say that I was doing things like riding the stationary bike for an hour, climbing the treadmill walking at incline for an hour (that was a butt kicker!), biking 30 miles on my real bike, doing cardio for 2 hours, lifting increasing amounts of weight. Cody kept me going each week with new exercises or at least increasing the amount of time or weight that he expected out of me with each training session.

With the sudden loss of five pounds my attitude improved as well. Miss Mojo appeared on occasion, checking in. Reaffirming that I was still committed to the goal, even though it was coming up fast! It was, after all, spring, and it was an early June wedding. It was gonna be close.

By April 8th, my weight was down to 184#! I hadn't seen that number in a long time!

I had just two more months to go and was feeling pretty stressed with the deadline looming. What else could I do to get faster results, I wondered? I really didn't want to cut my calories much more. I was hanging around 1,800 calories per day and felt I needed most of those to not be hungry. (Which really was a bunch of bunk. I was rarely physically hungry, I was *emotionally* hungry.) My average calories burned was around 2,500 per day. At that I was burning about 700 or so calories per day more than I was taking in. I was definitely

 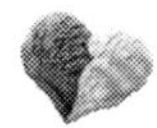

going in the right direction but I just wished I'd learned the magic all those months ago.

My last discovery was this: I tracked the calories burned on all the different cardio machines and learned that for me the rowing machine, stair stepper, and stationary bike all yielded about 350 calories burned per hour. But jogging, I was pleased to find out, burned closer to 700 per hour! Guess what I was going to focus on? You got it. Screw the other cardio exercises. I was going to focus on running. And, whenever possible, I was going to slip in a second workout in addition to my current routine. My knees would hold for a couple of months.

Miss Mojo said I could do this, and I believed her.

At the end of 5 weeks on the BodyBugg I was down ten pounds! I was 181#.

At the end of 7 weeks, I weighed 177#!

At the end of week 11, the day before the big wedding, I checked in at 167#!

From March 20 to June 4 I had lost 29#! Percent body fat was down from 40% to 28%

My measurements were as follows:

Chest : 36 - down 6 inches
Waist: 33 - down 7 inches
Hips: 43 - down 6 inches
Thighs: 18 - down 2 inches

Total inches lost: 21

Best part of all? I looked (and felt) HOT! And my little Miss Mojo was whooping and hollering all over the place! I really couldn't believe I'd pulled it off! And despite all the ups and downs I'd gone through.

Finally, comfortable with my final pre-wedding numbers, I went shopping for a hot Mother of the Bride dress and for the first time that I could remember, I not only didn't hate shopping, I loved it! I tried on dress after dress after dress until I found "the one." It was a softly clingy, just to the knee, sleeveless, bright red over the bodice and black from the bodice down number that clung in all the right places. It had a glittery, black jacket that sparkled under the lights. It screamed just the right amount of fashion, mixed with bling, on top of class. It was perfect. I couldn't wait to wear it.

The day before the wedding I showed up at the gym and asked Cody if someone could take our picture together, since he'd been such a huge influence in getting me there. I was hoping Bernie could have been there too but he was on vacation. But he had sent me congratulations from afar.

I showed up at Cody's desk dressed in my fancy new dress, barely able to contain myself I was so excited. And when he took one look at me (in something other than my workout clothes) he let out a huge whistle and called all the other trainers over to make a big fuss! I felt like I'd just won the Miss America pageant or something.

"You look amazing," he beamed at me. "Wow!" He took my hand and twirled me around as if we were on the dance floor. Then a couple of the other trainers joined in, as if taking turns to dance with a woman my age was a chance they shouldn't miss. They took a bunch of photos and then I said to Cody, "Wait here a sec. I'll be right back," and I disappeared off to the locker room.

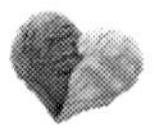

Miss Mojo was about as strong as she could possibly be. She'd been hinting at an idea for a few days before the photo shoot and I'd been sitting on the fence about it – until that moment. Cody didn't know what I was up to but when I walked back out into the gym in a very colorful bikini, he got everyone whooping and hollering again!

Cody had been right. Despite all those non-productive months that I thought had been a waste of time (not to mention, money), I had indeed been building muscle. Lots of muscle. In my legs. In my butt. Certainly in my arms. But, Baby, all those hundreds of ab workouts and crunches-upon-crunches sessions had most definitely paid off on my stomach. While it wasn't perfect, it was the flattest and the tightest I'd seen in a very long time and I was pleased as punch to show it off!

Of course, Cody had to bask in the glory as well. "Didn't I tell you to trust me?" He grinned ear to ear as the other trainers gathered around to congratulate us both, after we'd taken our fill of photos.

"Yes, you did. And I'm so glad I listened to you – and Bernie." I nodded to a couple of the trainers who had shaken my hand and given me pats on the back as they returned to their cubicles.

"You can't outrun the fork," he said.

"It's got two more legs than you," I replied. We laughed and hugged again.

"You really do look amazing. But does this mean you're done training, now that the big goal has been achieved?" He looked worried.

"Not a chance. I'm not done yet. I'd like to see just how much more I can lose since it's going so well. I'm at 167 now. Let's reassess at 160, how's that?"

"Sounds good. And I'll get the manager to put your story on the success board, so be sure to bring one of those bikini pictures when you get back from the wedding and you'll be another bright star on the walk of fame." He held up an imaginary camera and acted as though he was snapping me as if he were a photographer from the Paparazzi. "You're a star," he hollered, as I headed back to the locker room. And I felt like one. So did Miss Mojo.

***

The wedding was a huge success – at least after the rehearsal dinner. The venue was near Vail, Colorado at a place called Four Eagle Ranch. It was a beautiful old homestead that no longer raised cattle but still kept the country feel and history of a working ranch and now served as a backdrop for weddings and other such groups. This time of year the fields were filled with gorgeous flowers of many colors, popping like fireworks in nature's garden.

Tiny wooden cabins, many years old, peppered the property, as if the place had been a little town at one time. There were even horses and wagons and any number of beautiful antiques that reinforced the unique rustic and historic ambiance.

They had a magnificent backdrop of the Rocky Mountains and, all fingers crossed, if the weather went right, the photo ops should be spectacular. If not, there was an inner banquet hall in what was once a huge barn, which would certainly hold everyone. But the ambiance for a 3 p.m. wedding in the mountains, some still covered in snow on the 6th of June, was

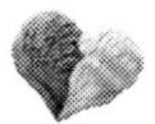

priceless. We were all saying a little prayer to the weather gods, as the forecast was a bit sketchy.

We met at the ranch Friday evening for all the rehearsal stuff. The weather, perfect. And after much checking off lists and double-checking details, it was time to grab some grub at the rehearsal dinner, which, in sticking with the ranch theme, was to be hot dogs and hamburgers and s'mores and all that went with that. We all headed to the hotel where we were all staying and prepared to head to the grilling area when the weather gods finally let go of their patience and it began to pelt us with a snow-rain mix.

If you're not familiar with mountain living, suffice it to say that anything can and will happen when it comes to the weather. A snow fall the first week of June was no rare event. Temperatures could drop to freezing by midnight and yet by noon be 70 degrees with all traces of snow melted, nearly as fast as it had come in. Since it was cold enough to snow, that meant that the temperature was at least 32 degrees or less, and few, if any folks, even thought about bringing or needing warm clothes.

Except me. I'm that odd duck that keeps a winter coat, mittens and a hat in my car year round because being cold to me is the cruelest form of torture on the planet. And was I glad I did. We all waited out the weather for an hour or so and, finally, the weather gods, having flexed their muscles to remind everyone just who was in charge after all, backed off the snow and rain just enough so that everyone finally ventured out of their rooms and the party began.

My first smiley moment happened when the maid of honor, Alexis, came up to me with a huge look of astonishment and said, "Holy cow, have you lost a bunch of weight or what, girl? Your jeans are like trying to fall off your butt!"

I grinned like a woman with a secret. "Yeah, I've been spending some time at the gym," I replied, as if losing nearly 30 pounds since she had seen me at the bridal shower a few months earlier was no big deal.

"Wow, you look amazing. How'd you do it? Weight Watchers or something?" I could tell she wasn't happy with her own weight and wished she too could magically snap her fingers and drop twenty pounds. "I just don't have time to do the gym, being in medical school," she bemoaned. "They don't give us time to breathe or sleep, much less work out."

"Well, the good news is that it's really 80 percent what you eat and only 20 percent exercise, " I shared. "If that helps any."

"Well, they barely give us time to eat either," she countered. "And I sure as hell don't have time to cook. Thus it's fast food day after day and you know just how good that is." She rolled her eyes. "Maybe some day, if I live through med school, I can give it a try. But you – she pointed her finger up and down at me, "You need to buy some new jeans, girl. Before these fall off of you!"

Miss Mojo was grinning to beat the band.

By morning the sun was out, the birds were singing, the snow was melting, and the weather forecast called for a beautiful day. Even the clouds stayed away so that the incredible mountain vista took center stage as backdrop for everything.

The wedding was perfect. Shaun was absolutely gorgeous in her sleek but simple satiny gown that spelled pure class. And little Dawson, age 7, looked so grown up in his tuxedo. And the happy couple?

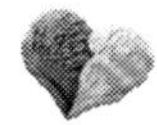

Well, I couldn't have been happier for them. They were obviously very much in love. And that's all one can wish for one's children.

As for me ... all was right with the world! For a while ...

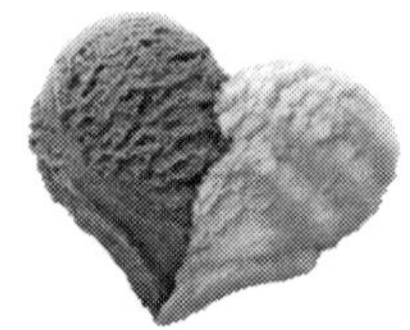

CHAPTER 17

Falling Apart

The wedding was behind me and I thought that I wouldn't be so focused on calories and workouts anymore. But no – it was almost the other way around. With my clothes getting looser and looser, my newest addiction seemed to be to see just how far I could go. I really didn't think I had much more room to go before my body would rebel and simply say no. They always say that, if your body thinks you might be starving it, it holds onto your weight even tighter. And so, as I mentioned to Cody, I thought 160 pounds sounded like it was doable.

So I kept my workout routine, just got rid of the two-a-days and the excessive running. Of course, in the weeks I'd been pounding my body so hard I'd had many a day with pain. A sore shoulder here, a tight sciatic nerve there. My aching back that had been a giant pain for years. And both of my knees, pretty messed up since way back. I just got used to some of it. This getting older crap was definitely not for the faint of heart!

I had especially noticed a couple of things which, now that I had the time, I gave myself the license to look into. The first was a horrible sciatic pain that would shoot from just under my butt cheek all the way down the back of my right thigh to the back of my knee. The only way I could describe that unique pain is being like what it must be like if you put your finger into an electrical socket. It felt shocking! If you've ever touched an electric fence or gotten shocked in some way, you know what I mean. I noticed that it tended to happen after a certain exercise or two, so I dropped those two from my routine and it seemed to simmer down, at least somewhat.

The other oddity was that for all the weight lifting I'd been doing for all those months (nothing excessively,) my left hand seemed to be unhappy for some reason and responded by suddenly feeling weak. Just turning the nob on the door and pulling it to open took much more effort than usual. I couldn't think of any pulls or injuries to it, but there it was. It also seemed to pick up a slight tremor in it, that was new.

I reported these two things to Cody and he wasn't sure what to make about the situation either, but suggested I take a couple of days off completely and just let my body rest. It was obviously trying to tell me something. Likely I'd pinched a nerve or something.

And so I did. I spent a few days completely relaxing, just soaking in the hot tub and even got a fabulous 90-minute massage from my favorite massage guy, Ira, who I'd been seeing once a month for over a year.

"What have you been doing differently?" he queried me. "You're usually tight but you're way more than that the last couple of times you've been in."

"I wish I knew," I replied. "It's killing me."

As he dug his hands into my oh-so-tight hamstring he asked, "Has he got you doing something different, lately?" (I think Ira was always looking out for me and was worried that Cody was over-working me.)

I shook my head and groaned. Not a good groan. One that said, please stop right now, as he tried to get the knots to loosen up. We discussed a variety of things to try, from Icy Hot patches to a heating pad, to straight ice, to stretches. I even added in a couple of extra massages over the next couple of weeks but the hamstring pain only seemed to be growing and the hand showed no intention of improving its weak sister behavior.

This went on for several months. Things would improve for a while then, for no apparent reason that damned hamstring would start screaming at me, sometimes so bad that I was limping. And in case I'd pinched a nerve, Cody had me pull a couple more exercises out of the line-up to see if that might help. But no luck.

My weight was still gradually dropping despite this frustration. I was down to about 160 pounds – the goal I'd set for myself after the wedding. I was still gradually losing, mostly by cutting my food down, since I wasn't keeping up the exercise level I had been at. I eventually leveled out at about 155.

I was thrilled to death with my weight loss success and how strong and fit I was. It had been since high school that I'd even come close to looking like that. I had pulled my favorite skinny jeans out of the back of the closet, dusted them off, and slid them on as if they were an old friend come to dinner! I was so glad I'd kept them. They were my ongoing motivation.

And of course, people at the gym were constantly complimenting me about my hard work. One trainer, who had been gone for many months, was totally shocked by my changes when he first saw me. He couldn't believe it. Bernie was always checking in with me and still would ask every week, "How's it going? And how's the food?" He wasn't going to let me slip after coming that far.

But as the pain didn't quit, I decided it was time to see someone. There was a new chiropractor in the neighborhood, Dr. Neal Nelson, and he'd sent out mailers to drum up some business. I decided to check him out. He was a young, energetic guy, passionate about his work. Kind of on the short side for a man, but his energy and bright blue eyes set me at ease right away. After I gave him my entire history and him giving me a full check-up, top to bottom, he said he'd rather I get an x-ray of my spine before he did anything. So he sent me on my way to a radiology clinic.

The long and the short of it was that the x-ray showed that not only did I have an extra vertebrae in my lower back (fairly rare, although not a problem, in and of itself), my back was a huge mess. So much so that Dr. Nelson suggested I see a spinal surgeon instead.

I was in shock. Sure, I'd had trouble with my back most of my life, especially for as many times as some horse or other dumped me off onto the hard ground. But spine surgery? I wasn't ready for that.

And so, I popped all the Advil I could take and went into a state of denial like so many people do when they receive information they don't want to hear. I told Cody what I had found out and suggested I just really lay low on the heavy workouts for a while. Perhaps just work in the pool for a bit, and see how things went from there. He agreed. It would be good for my knees as well.

Weeks went by and not only did things not improve, they kept getting worse. I was down to just water-walking – not even swimming – and the pain finally got to a point where something had to give. I couldn't take it any more.

Honestly, if I knew what the next couple of years had in store for me, I think I'd have ended it all right there.

Of course, I'd filled my daughter in about my back pain, but she was in Columbia, Missouri working on her orthopedic surgery residency and I hadn't seen her since the wedding. But luckily for me, she invited me out to spend Christmas with them. Lucky, not only because I would get to celebrate the holiday with them, but lucky because when she took one look at how badly I was limping by then, and how obvious my pain was – just bending over trying to put my shoes on was pure torture – she was on the phone to her boss, begging him to see me immediately.

And so, at 7:30 the following morning I met her teacher, Dr. Sloan, a spinal surgeon, and thanked God that sometimes it pays to know someone in the medical world. I suspect his usual wait time to get in for an appointment was likely several weeks and I'd surely be insane if I had to wait that long. His calm bedside manner helped simmer my terrified mind. But not completely

I suspected he was in his 50's; he was medium build, sort of swallowed up by his white lab coat with the pockets jammed full of the tools of his trade. It was easy to see that he was a man of much experience, as he put me through a variety of tests – reach this way, bend that way, can you touch your toes – that kind of thing. He scratched his bald head, in thought, then he shared with us how he couldn't diagnose anything without an MRI but based on what he saw and my history, he suspected I had some kind of pressure on my

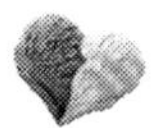

spinal cord that would need to be taken care of surgically, as soon as possible.

He'd gone through residency with a guy named Gary Ghiselli, who had gone on to set up practice in Denver. He recommended him highly and suggested I see him absolutely ASAP. That word, surgery, was rearing its ugly head again.

I was in shock. I had thought perhaps a pinched nerve or something. But surgery? Oh, my God.

The MRI proved what Dr. Sloan had suspected; my spinal cord was being compressed in several places, which is what was causing the pain. However, I couldn't entirely blame my active life style and years falling off horses for the situation. Apparently I had been born with spinal stenosis; and over the years the space inside my spinal canal where my spinal cord and nerves lived, had gotten tighter and tighter, leading up to the pain, which had reached excruciating levels at times. One day had been so bad that I needed Ira to help me get dressed after a massage, as I couldn't lift my leg enough at that point to climb into my pants.

All the while this was going on, my misbehaving left hand was getting worse as well. Dr. Ghiselli suggested we get an MRI of my neck, just in case there was stenosis there as well, compressing a nerve in my neck, which could be causing the weakness and tremor. And when these MRI results came back, everyone really got hot and bothered. Apparently my first MRI that had been plenty bad enough didn't hold a candle to the mess inside my neck. I believe they would have liked to repair the neck first and do the lower back later but as the tremor and weakness in my hand were annoying, they weren't part of my pain. That had to be fixed first.

So, we lined up not one, but two surgeries, one in February and one in April. The lower back first – which was a bugger in and of itself – then the neck, which involved two parts. First, lying on my back, they cut into my neck and moved my esophagus and trachea to get to my spine. After extensive work on that side, they put everything back in place, stitched me up, then turned me over (while still under anesthesia) and then sliced open the back side of my neck and worked on that for a while, fusing my neck vertebrae into one unit that would no longer bend as it once did. The whole point of which was to make it stronger and to keep my spinal cord from being crushed.

It was a killer surgery that had me in really rough shape for the first two weeks or so. Swallowing was terrible and I choked on meds several times per day.

I had to wear this huge, rigid neck brace around the clock for several weeks. Sleeping with that was a bugger.

I was so grateful for Shaun making the trip for both surgeries. She even slept in my hospital room and was so great staying on top of my care. She could only cut class like this for a few days and when she left she handed me over to my sister, Barb, who nursed me at her house for several days. I don't know where I would have been without these guys.

The good news post-surgeries was that the sciatic pain was mostly gone in a matter of days. That, in itself, was such a blessing. It didn't matter that I had to walk with a walker for weeks, couldn't drive for quite a while, and slowly moved from a cane to regular walking again – just losing that ungodly electric shooting jolt down the back of my leg was worth everything I had to go through to get there.

The not so great news items:

First, a few days after the back surgery I felt something shift in my back and that new something would result in a new groin pain, which, after several months again of hoping it would heal on its own, landed me back on the OR table in June before it simmered down.

Yet, one of the most shocking things that came out of nowhere and hit me over the head, completely rocking my world, was that damned left hand. Based on the MRI and my weakness/tremor symptoms, Dr. G was pretty confident that the neck surgery would likely take care of the unwanted symptoms. And for a short time post-op, the strength seemed to improve somewhat. But the symptoms never completely went away and just kept hanging around, driving me nuts!

At last Dr. G suggested I see a neurologist. He'd run out of ideas.

And so, I was on to the next doctor, who was stumped. Then finally to one who diagnosed me in a heartbeat – Dr. Mark Triehoft – who tried to tell me in his most supportive and empathetic way possible, that I had Parkinson's disease.

"That can't be possible," I resisted the news. "That's something old people get and I'm not old yet. Right?" At this point I was only in my early fifties. I begged God to tell me that this man was making a serious mistake.

I had experience with two people in my life with Parkinson's – my father, who also had Alzheimer's, and a man my mother worked for back in the 1960's, when they didn't have many drugs yet to minimize the tremors. As such, he was shaking and quaking all over the place all the time, and as a girl of about 10 or 12, his behavior scared me to death. Was my life going to look like that?

Dr. Triehoft put his hand gently on my shoulder. "First of all, this is not a death sentence. And secondly, you are in the very early stages. And in most patients, it tends to move relatively slowly, especially if you make exercise a big part of your lifestyle." He knew how hard it was for me to hear this. "No one seems to know why, but exercise seems to slow it down somehow."

I was sure that my face must have looked like someone had hit me over the head with a baseball bat. This just couldn't be happening to me ... not with all I had already been dealing with. My body was still trying to rehab after three major surgeries. Now this? Why me, God?

Dr. Triehoft continued filling my head with facts and figures about meds, symptoms to watch for, how often I should see him, and so much more but I was in a trance; I was numb. I heard very little.

What I did hear was this was a degenerative disease, meaning it would never get better, only worse. There was no cure. There were several drugs on the market and, while they generally helped with the tremors, some had bad side effects in and of themselves. The best the meds could do was just try to stay ahead of the symptoms. Some of which were not so great – rather like the left-handed weakness and tremor. Little did I know there were so many other possible symptoms that would likely show up as the disease progressed, such as balance issues, changes in my voice (that sucks being a speaker), extreme fatigue, changes in cognition, changes in facial expression which can make someone appear as though they are angry or not paying attention. The list goes on. In fact, it is often called a "snowflake disease" because no two patients have the exact same symptoms.

I cried all the way home, driving through the tears once again.

It took me a long time to get used to this label. In fact, I kept it a secret from almost everyone for nearly three years. All I could think of was that I was still single and out there in the dating world. Who was going to want a girlfriend with Parkinson's? As one guy told me, it's one thing to have a mate of many years come down with something like that, whether a disease or illness or pace maker, or whatever. It was quite another thing to elect to date someone with such a liability. Yep – he pretty much confirmed just what I had been thinking.

The good thing was that I got connected to a young-onset Parkinson's group in the Denver area where at least I didn't feel alone. These were not the typical people that usually depict the face of Parkinson's: the little old man or lady, all hunched over, shuffling around and shaking uncontrollably.

No, these were much younger-than-usual folks who had been dealing with the illness for years. I met a young woman in her 30's with a couple of little kids who seemed to be carrying on just fine. There were several people in their 40's and even one young gal in her 20's who was newly diagnosed and still reeling with the news. And there were quite a number in their 50's. Most were doing OK and only a few were as jumpy as Michael J. Fox, at least how he's seen on TV. Of course, he's been fighting Parkinson's for 20-plus years, so is certainly farther down the road than many of us, and his symptoms make that obvious.

All in all, once the diagnosis was made, all my symptoms made perfect sense.

It just wasn't what I wanted to hear.

Over time, I've been able to make a little peace with my illness, at least as best I can. Partly I realize that so many of us have something we don't wish we had. From cancer to diabetes, to heart disease, to multiple sclerosis, to having to go to dialysis three times per week. None of us get out of this world totally Scott-free. There are a lot more things that I would have been even more unhappy with.

To end 2011 with even more fun and excitement, my knees had kept their screaming up as well. They just didn't scream as loud as everything else had. They'd been bone-on-bone for some time and if I got them fixed before the end of the year, I would save $10,000 on my insurance. That was a no-brainer. So I told them to go ahead and do the replacements, and in October I had one knee done and the other in November.

Just call me bionic. I only wished I moved as well as all the TV bionic people!

I was looking for 2012 being a new year that would let me get my body back in at least civil shape again. I didn't *have* to be as fit as I was. I just had to keep moving, both to keep my weight in line and stave off Parkinson's. My back wasn't perfect; it was only moderately uncomfortable for the most part, with a flare-up here and there. With everything I'd gone through, my weight had wandered back into the 180's again.

The good news was that I had met someone! His name was George and we met online. We hit it off instantly and in fact, I first met him the day before my second knee surgery on 11/11/11. A day that's supposed to be a lucky day. Just ask all the folks who got married on that day for that very reason.

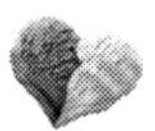

He'd been a paramedic in his younger years and had his own health issues he'd dealt with for a long time, so my stuff didn't chase him away and his stuff didn't bother me. And we could talk medicine and both of us understood what was being talked about.

I was staying at Mary Ann's house post-op this time and George even came over one night and brought a pizza for us. Miss Mojo, who had laid low for so long while I was really a mess of healing, actually peeked her nose out and reminded me to watch what I was eating with a new man in my life. So at least that was an incentive to move a bit faster. I increased my water walking to an hour nearly every day. More importantly, as always, a little romance always got me happy and happiness didn't send me out as often for a sugar fix.

Then the next crisis fell. My mom had been living in a senior's home and she'd taken a fall and ended up in the hospital. For the better part of two months I sat with her, often sleeping on the bunk in her room. I certainly didn't make it to the gym and I lived on hospital food. It was a very tough time for her. She was in a lot of pain a lot of the time. Which I could now relate to. The stress of worrying about her took its toll on me and I ate to fill the unhappiness. After 2-1/2 months she passed away. By the time we'd taken her back to Wisconsin for the funeral and burial, we were all emotionally and physically exhausted. We came home and crashed for days.

One night, months later, I was sound asleep in bed when I was awakened with a jolt to the sound of someone screaming. No, more like shrieking, as if in terrible pain. Honestly, it sounded like someone was being burned at the stake. I live alone and was wondering who could possibly be screaming in my house, when suddenly, I realized it was me! I was screaming at the top of my lungs, out of sheer pain! Horrible, intense, excruciating pain! I suddenly felt like I must be in the hands of the Taliban or ISIS and was being tortured to death.

As I went to move in bed to see what the hell was happening I was jolted with yet another blaze of fire shooting through my system. It was that horrible electrical, my-back's-on-fire, this must be what it's like to be electrocuted sensation coursing through me. I screamed again, and again, and again. Non-stop. It literally took my breath away. But there was no one to hear me.

I figured out pretty quickly that the pain stopped if I stopped moving – even an inch, in any direction. But forget that crucial fact and the taser would return instantly and punishingly.

What to do? It was 5:45 a.m. on a Sunday. Fortunately I always kept my cell phone on the headboard, so if I could reach it, I could at least call for help. I slowly reached for my cell and got jolted with that cattle prod sensation again, pulsing through my entire body. Holy crap. I gritted my teeth and still screamed as I reached for and grabbed the phone. After trying several friends (most turned off their phones at night) I finally reached my sister to come help. She only lived a few minutes away and by the time she'd arrived I'd been on the phone with Dr. G, who told me to get to the ER as fast as possible. Needless to say, I was terrified at the idea of anyone touching me – paramedics or otherwise – for fear of the cattle prod again. So I had my sister rustle up one of my rarely used pain pills and we found a single, incredible Valium tucked way in the back of my medicine chest, leftover from some MRI or other I'd had during the year. Once I downed them and they had a few minutes to kick in, I was able to get into the car with help and spent the afternoon getting intravenous Valium and Dilaudid to help with the pain. Three days later another surgery was performed on my back during which it was discovered that I'd had a cyst within my spine that had ruptured, "traumatically," as they described it. (I'll say).

And once again I was back to walking with a walker, back on pain meds, back to physical therapy. As I said earlier, had I known what was coming over those couple of years, I think I just would have checked out instead.

They say that God only gives you as much as you can handle but honestly, I didn't believe it any more.

For all that I'd been through, I was grateful that my weight had held pretty well around 185. Not great, but could be so much worse. I was finally able to get back to the gym where I spent a lot of time just walking in the water. After several weeks I was able to lead my dating classes again, take on some coaching clients, do some writing, and even take a trip with George to Cozumel several months after the craziness had finally simmered down. It was so much fun to share the island with him and see him learn to dive. We had some pretty good times together for a year or so, but unfortunately, our relationship was not to last. And we said good-bye, yet still remained friends.

At last my body seemed to settle down to a dull roar. I'd come to the conclusion that my back was never going to be pain free, but I've learned how to handle most of its arguing with me with various combinations of Advil, Tylenol, massage, and on rare occasions, a pain pill. I continued to come to grips with the Parkinson's situation. I don't keep it a secret any more. My mantra is, "I may have Parkinson's but it doesn't have me." Otherwise I'd have likely made myself crazy before now.

But my weight was getting close to 190 again. And with it, my attitude went in the crapper. I'd struggled with depression for so long, I had a hard time just getting out of bed every day. My mom had been gone for two years by then and I missed her every day. I was in a deep, dark funk and couldn't see any way out. I had to do something different.

As for Miss Mojo – I hadn't seen her in months.

I pulled out a jar of peanut butter and a spoon and prayed for some relief in the heavenly, sticky substance that would melt on my tongue.

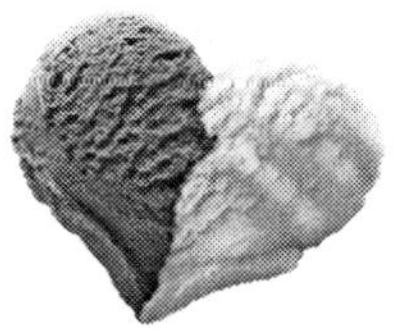

CHAPTER 18

Going To The Fat Farm

Most people have amazing vacation locations on their Bucket List: Tahiti, Iceland, China, for instance.

I have had something more unusual on mine for years; I've always wanted to attend a Fat Farm. At least that's what they used to call them. Nowadays that's politically incorrect. Today they are more likely called Fitness Boot Camps, although that can still be a bit unclear since the military still uses the term boot-camp to imply the first six weeks of basic training, where young, already in-shape men and women suddenly get even fitter than their twenty-something bodies could imagine.

With the popularity of reality TV shows like the *Biggest Loser*, more and more people are considering such remedies, looking to find that magic pill that will help them almost instantly shed pounds and change their lives in some fancy resort location far from the madding crowd and all the temptations of the real world.

Furthermore, many people imagine attending a boot camp as a way to control what goes in their mouths and bodies. They want someone to keep food under lock and key for them so they can't get at it, no matter how much begging they do. And after a given amount of time with someone else in control of their food decisions, combined with some ridiculously amazing number of hours working out, they imagine that they will somehow return to their old high school selves from 20, 30, or more years ago with flat tummies, taut tushies, and the toned arms of a weight lifter. After all, it happens on the *Biggest Loser* all the time, so it must be true. Right?

Honestly, it was amazing that my body hadn't rebelled long before now! In fact, it had been rioting in other ways, I just hadn't really put two and two together in quite this way before. I had fought mild depression for the last several years … enough so that I'd been on anti-depressants for some time. And since my mom's passing just two years before, I was still struggling with all that went with that.

Family members and I had stayed by her bedside for much of her last two months before she passed away, which I was grateful for. Yet the emotional exhaustion that went along with that had definitely taken its toll on my own health as well. Plus, of course, she wasn't there to talk to anymore and I kept reaching for the phone to call her and about the time I could feel the phone in my hand, reality would hit. She would never be there again. And then the tears would come. Even two years later.

On top of the depression I tired easily. Needed a nap every afternoon. My energy sucked. My motivation to do anything sucked even more. I hadn't put out any new blogs or books or much of anything for a long time either, and that's really bad because, believe it or not, these writing projects are usually

 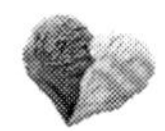

what kick-start me into my Energizer Bunny mode. It's like I tell folks who ooohhh and aahhhh that I'm an author: writing for me is not a punishment. Rather, it's like the reward I get for getting all my other stuff done. I GET to go write. But that side of me had seemingly taken a vacation of its own.

I really, REALLY needed to take better care of my body. I knew that. I wasn't a young pup any more and if I didn't want to be trapped in the rocking chair early, it seemed obvious that I'd better do something serious and soon. I was ever-so fortunate that I wasn't battling diabetes, high blood pressure, heart disease, and all the other fun stuff that just seems to come on the road to getting older. But all those orthopedic surgeries I'd undergone had not turned my body into some bionic wonder, as in the olden days of the Six Million Dollar Man (or woman, in this case.)

Instead, while they had improved many issues involving pain, (back pain, knee pain, neck pain, etc.) those new joints were simply not my own and, while they kept me going pretty well, I always knew they weren't the ones I was born with. They simply didn't allow me to do many of the things I used to.

I considered my bucket list again ... hiking in Iceland or walking the Great Wall of China or SCUBA diving in Pilau (can't wait for that one!) all demanded that I get this body in the best shape I could, WHILE I STILL COULD.

And so, during a bout of feeling sorry for myself and doing my best to stave off depression once again, I Googled "Fat Farm." And in just a few minutes and a few clicks on my keyboard, I was registered to attend my own boot camp in a couple of weeks at Rancho Cortez, Dude Ranch and Fitness

Ranch in the heart of the Hill Country of Texas, a bit over an hour's drive from San Antonio.

How did I settle on this particular place? Mostly the price was right. I'd actually checked on rates for Fitness Ranches before and it seemed like three to five thousand bucks per week was about par. This one had several a la cart program possibilities but the one that caught my eye was the two-week Boot Camp at about $2,000. It proved to be a dirt cheap program where you share sleeping space in a bunkhouse with other el-cheapo's like me. There were also private rooms or double rooms available for those folks with more moolah to spend and a driving need for privacy and a decent mattress.

The photos of the facilities made the place look quite simple, and it was. Looking over their web site I noted that there were not even any fancy exercise machines in the gym. This place was back to basics and touted hiking in the great outdoors, water aerobics, low calorie food, a campfire at the end of the day, and yep – you could even ride a horse if you'd a mind to.

The schedule they had posted on the website looked a bit daunting but I wasn't horribly worried about the workouts, actually. I was pretty good about getting in at least 30 minutes of something aerobic a few days a week and a 15-minute course of twice weekly puttering around with free weights. And while I was pretty curious just how far I could push my body with the multiple workouts per day, I was most concerned about how my body would handle the likely withdrawal of being cut off from my usual unhealthy menu, which I was certain wasn't going to be served up at mealtime while I was there.

 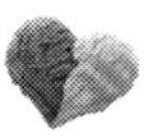

I was especially excited about the idea that all food would be under lock and key and, not having a car during my stint there, combined with the fact that the closest town was reportedly 20 or 30 minutes away as the crow flies, would severely limit my favorite high fructose corn syrup favorites from showing up anytime soon. I wondered if there were tasty treats lying around somewhere for the dudes. There had to be, right? But I imagined it would be a bit hard to wander into the dining hall looking nonchalant and innocent, then steal some junk food when the kitchen help wasn't watching. But, my evil side reminded me that there were always possibilities, if one wanted it badly enough. After all, I'm a closet sugar addict. I knew how to hide my addiction from others at the same time that I got my fix filled!

Dammit! Here I was anticipating behaving badly already and I wasn't even there yet! "Wake up!" I shouted at myself as I turned to the photos of folks on their web pages happily working out. I wondered how much they had to pay them to smile like that?

They also had posted a bunch of testimonials from past attendees, which caught my eye. Some from various places around the world. (Now that was impressive.)

My goals in going there were ...

***

First, I needed a swift kick in the butt and someone to drive me (metaphorically speaking) for two solid weeks. I needed some firm expectations and boundaries. And someone with a cattle prod who would be willing to use it on me to get me zapped back to life. It sounded better than a defibrillator shocking me back to life, half-naked in some emergency room, which was certainly a possibility if I let things get worse.

Second, I knew that I needed to have my food doled out to me. No excuses. No cheating. My poor body would likely go into shock being fed healthy food for the first time in years. I was eager to see just how it felt when given something besides ice cream, popcorn, and fudge as staples.

Third, I wanted to learn how to work within the confines of a specific schedule. A routine. What a concept. As a writer who works at home whenever the mood struck, I really craved structure for a change. If I could learn structure I bet I could actually get some things done.

And lastly, I wanted to lose some serious weight! If I could lose 10 pounds in two weeks I would be amazed and thrilled. It was a lofty goal but I desperately wanted to see that scale drop below 160 pounds for the first time in many years. Of course keeping it off when I got home would be another story, but if I could just get this damned kick-start here, I was convinced that it would surely give me an edge I hadn't seemed to be able to conjure up on my own.

This was it. No turning back. I sat down at my computer and began the process of filling out my application

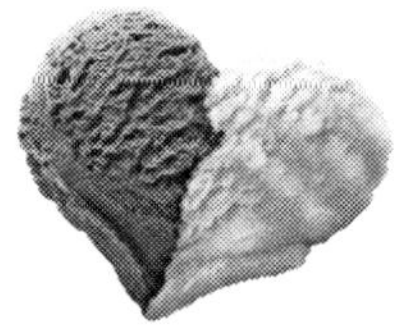

CHAPTER 19

Hot, Hot, Hot

We arrived on Sunday, as the sun pounded down on us in the hottest part of the day. (Note to self: if I ever do this again, I promise, I'll take the red-eye flight in the middle of the night if it means that I wouldn't need to be out in this Devil's oven at the peak temperature of the day.) Honestly, it must have been like 105 degrees. "Welcome to the desert!" I felt it say to me. "Hope you like to sweat." I instinctively wiped my brow – which would be the first of a zillion times during my stay.

The van driver, a stocky Latino man named Raul who picked us up (myself and another boot camp attendee named Jim) at the San Antonio airport, explained that he would drive us about 75 miles through the empty, desert-like Texas Hill Country (aptly named) before we would finally reach the ranch. "So sit back and enjoy the ride," he grinned. I wasn't sure if he was grinning just to be polite, or if he was laughing his ass off at the next unsuspecting motley crew (us) who had really no idea what we had gotten ourselves into. And not to mention, were doling out 2,000 fine American dollars to do so as well!

Jim was 50 something, with salt and pepper hair and a quiet demeanor. Since I sat in the back, he and the driver seemed to strike up a conversation and I took in the landscape. The land was dry and rocky and peppered with squatty little juniper trees. The pale blue sky was loaded with puffy clouds and a sun so hot it seemed that it would fry your skin off in a heartbeat, with or without sunscreen. (Note to self: Apply sunscreen every hour for the next two weeks! And make sure the SPF is 50+!)

The barren landscape went on as far as the eye could see, with only an occasional teeny, tiny town that we rolled into and out of in under two minutes. Not much in any of them except for one ancient gas station that also served burgers and hot dogs, plus a few small grocery must-haves like bread and milk. It also doubled as the town's post office.

I couldn't imagine breaking down in my car out there somewhere. Or what about the cowboys and pioneers of old trudging along some barely-there trail in this scorching heat with a huge herd of cattle they were moving for many miles? If jeans and long sleeved shirts, boots and chaps weren't hot enough for the men of the day, for any women who tagged along, they'd likely be wearing huge, long skirts that would only hasten their dehydration factor. No wonder life was short back then. Probably even shorter if you were a wee one.

I questioned myself for a moment – I was pretty sure that the ranch's website had boasted air conditioning. Right? I shook the thought out of my mind, but still felt huge empathy for our ancestors who had made this empty place a home.

At last we arrived at the fancy gate that said Rancho Cortez. The first impression of the place was all cowboy, from

 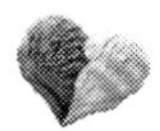

the brass figure of a full-sized cowboy leaning on the fence post at the entry way, to the strategically placed aloe plants that lined the long driveway up to the main buildings. The place was rather sprawly, with several cabins scattered across the gentle hillside. Not a soul was in sight – anywhere. Hmmmm, I wondered. Should I be worried? Naw – likely they were inside hugging their air conditioners.

"Here we are," Raul pointed out the obvious. "You can walk over to the office to officially check in, after you put your things away, OK?" While we were prepared for our bunkhouse accommodations, I think we were both still a bit shocked by, shall we say, the "rustic reality" of it all!

"Well, I'm not planning to do more than sleep here," I said to Jim, a bit nervously. "No need for something fancy if that's the case." With the driver nearby, Jim only gave me a look that said, "Hope you're right," and we left it at that.

The bunkhouse was exactly what you might envision in an army boot camp. There were 15 cots in the gals' side. I assume something similar on the boys' side. Most were bunk beds. I chose the only single bed that didn't have an upper bunk. The floor and walls were plywood. There were two bathrooms – only one had a mirror, if you want to call it that. It was akin to the mirrors at the House of Mirrors attraction at a carnival and only filled part of the space over the sink. Want to check your full image? I guessed you'd have to go to the gym, where per usual, mirrors likely lined the walls to help folks check their form, and anything else a gym rat needed to look at.

There was no light over the sink so I realized that taking my contacts in and out would be a bit tricky and would have to be done out in the bedroom area. The downside to that is they are easier to lose. I did have a back-up pair.

I had already heard there were only two gals in the bunkhouse, fortunately, so we'd be able to spread out a bit. Thank God for small favors.

As I took in my living space for the next two weeks I reminded myself that I came here for the boot camp atmosphere and to save bucks, and I confirmed with myself that I wouldn't be spending much time in my bedroom anyway. So why not just think of it as Girl Scout Camp and leave it at that?

According to Google, the ranch was unique in that it was half Dude Ranch and half Fitness Ranch. And the website described how this unique mix seemed to work out just fine. The cowboy/horsie/dude folks tended to hang out around the barns, activity building, or the campfire after dark. The exercise nuts in the gym, the indoor pool, or the fitness lounge. At mealtimes, everyone shared the cozy, intimate mess hall but rarely saw each other the rest of the day.

And while everything did look pretty rustic, all appeared clean, well kept, and organized. A good sign, I thought.

Original shock behind us, I headed for the office to get checked in.

Jim opened the squeaky screen door for me and held it as I walked in first. The 10 foot by 8 foot office was old but cozy, and smelled like a blend of tobacco, sweat, horses, leather, and potato chips. Every square inch of wall and table/desk space was filled with cowboy paraphernalia. Framed newspaper articles, many about the owner, Larry Cortez, in his younger years as a successful rodeo cowboy. Ribbons from horse shows. Old cowboys hats and fancy spurs. It was everything I'd imagined it would be, only dustier.

Then I noticed the one small area with various items for sale including water bottles, T-shirts with Rancho Cortez emblazoned on the front, sunscreen, bug spray and of course you guessed it ... snacks! I'm talking candy bars, Fritos, mixed nuts, and God knows what else. I was afraid to look! Dammit! Just knowing they were this close was torture. Maybe that was part of the program? Test your willpower from the get-go? Naw. I remembered that it wasn't just a fitness camp. There would be real people here too who had every right to partake. It wasn't their problem that I felt better with all such temptations under lock and key!

A 50-something, slender cow-gal behind the counter had a grin that would make anyone feel at home. Her faded Wrangler jeans and rough-out cowboy boots reflected years of use but they still fit her like a glove. "You must be Mary Jo and Jim," she smiled that smile at us, making us feel comfy in what could otherwise have been seen as a strange and daunting place. I wondered how she knew who we were, after all, we hadn't been required to send a photo and I assumed there were other attendees due in as well – at least that was my impression. (I found out later that we were the last two due in, so it was a no-brainer.)

"I'm Cheryl, and I'll give you two the scoop on everything, from the lay of the land, to when and where the group will be meeting before dinner, what time meals are served, etc." She went through her dog and pony show, and answered our remaining questions (which she always lead off with a "Yes, Ma'am or No, Sir"). It didn't take me long to realize that was just the norm here. I would hear those phrases repeated at least once in almost any conversation for my entire stay. I didn't mind. I've always thought that there was something to be said for a little politeness and Southern hospitality.

About the time Cheryl had finished her canned speech about the place and then let us know what time Michael, the head trainer, wanted to meet with us after dinner, Jim and I realized it was probably time to pay up. As he went digging for his wallet and I pulled my credit card out of my pocket and held it out for Cheryl to get the ball rolling, I was surprised when she said, "You might want to hang on to those for now. At least until morning. Just in case you change your mind ... or something."

I think what she meant was, "Just in case you really don't appreciate what it is you're getting into here, we give you the night to sleep on it before we take your money!" (Apparently over the years some folks got cold feet and bugged out mucho pronto once they realized they weren't going for two weeks of fun in the sun in Hawaii or something. And it was likely easier not to have charged them beforehand than to refund them later. Cheryl looked to us to see which way we might slide.

Jim and I, however, both took a leap of faith and paid her on the spot. There was no turning back now. My $2,000 had been paid and I was ready for whatever they threw at me. Or so I thought.

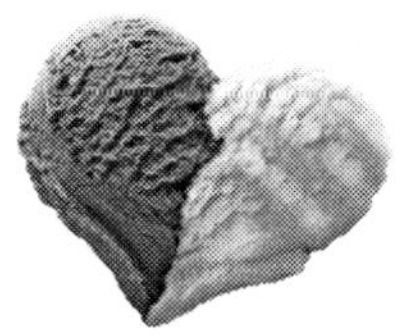

CHAPTER 20

Let The Games Begin!

According to Cheryl, our trainer, Michael Rivera, wanted us all in the lounge at 5 p.m. to start things off – I assumed the usual things like weigh-in, expectations, getting to know one another. Welcome party, so to speak. I certainly didn't expect we'd be working out the evening of our arrival, but I was about to learn differently right quick.

I wandered in promptly at 5, but was surprised to find myself one of only four obvious participants awaiting our fate. Was that it? Only four of us for the next two weeks? I felt mixed. As in, what the hell is wrong with this place that there are only four of us suckers? (Sure didn't look like the website with all the happy workout faces.) Or else – were we blessed with so few people here that we got amazing, nearly one-on-one coaching?

I actually learned much later that most people are smart enough to avoid the hill country of Texas in the heat of August – especially considering that outdoor hikes were part of the promised activities. My need to get away and my desperation for a quick kick in the butt hadn't lead me to checking out such details as what was the high temperature (mid 90's with super heavy humidity) for this region during the heat of the day in Texas? In other words, the fault was mine. Smart people simply didn't go there during the hottest month of the year. Duh.

About that time, in zoomed Michael. His arrival reminded me of the Road Runner cartoons, where this blur of energy, smoke, speed, and power arrives in like a whirling dervish, all happening so fast that no one knows exactly what just happened! The only thing missing was the, "Beep, Beep!" By the time the dust settled from his entrance I knew things were looking up.

If I was going to beat myself up for two weeks, the least thing God could give me was some decent scenery to admire. I'm not talking about the foreboding desert-like landscape. I'm talking about Michael. He's probably late 20-something, 5'6", and 160 pounds of solid muscle with a huge smile and a twinkle in his eye. He's Latino by background, dons the facial hair that's popular today – just a small sliver on his chin, and hair cut short and gelled just enough to slick it back fashionably. His arms bulge with smooth muscles that show years of work, no steroids needed. He filled out his workout pants to a T, with the lines of his derriere as well as thighs and calves quite pleasantly evident as well. He was the epitome of fitness but with a smile – not the grouchy demeanor of many who work equally hard to manufacture such a body and then gloat in showing it off to the lesser folks who could never aspire to such a feat.

He was going to be my trainer (and eye candy) for the next two weeks! Ahhhhh! Thank you, Jesus! If for no other reason than that, my $2,000 has already been well spent!

 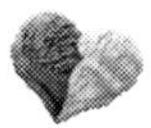

It was obvious that Michael drives the program. He's passionate about teaching people about fitness. His energy is of the Energizer Bunny variety – rarely stopping to sit or stand still. As if he can't wait for whatever exciting thing might come along at any second. My mom used to call that having "ants in your pants," but for Michael it was just his auto-pilot.

"Hey, guys. Welcome, welcome, welcome," he looked to each of us with the look that said, "No worries. You can trust me." And we did. He was infectious. And if we could return home after two weeks with only ten percent of what he was, we'd all be huge successes.

He opened a file folder that he carried and perused his notes and info. Glancing at each of us as he flipped through the pages, he identified everyone – both for himself and for the group.

Who were we?

Here's a summary of all my fellow plebes ...

Carol, 27, a customer service rep who lives in Houston, is the heaviest with about 100 pounds to lose. She, like Michael, is a bundle of energy. She proves to be like a short Chatty Kathy social director, jumping in to help with whatever's needed whenever it's needed.

She was once a cross-country runner in high school, so she hadn't always been heavy, but seemed to balloon up in college, where in her senior year she had the horrible realization that she'd taken the wrong direction in her education and suddenly knew in her heart that she really wanted to be a nurse. She just didn't know it until the end of her education was on the horizon. Then, she didn't know what to do. She was preparing to go back to school part time and just knew she had to do something with her weight while she was at it.

Turned out that she was also a techno-nerd: the go-to person when anyone needed computer help downloading something or transferring photos or anything else that came along. She became an amazing asset to the group. And she had signed on for a month. She, like all of us, has tried a variety of diets but had just never found the magic pill.

Chris, 43, tall, blue-eyed, and sandy-haired was once in the Army. Back in the day, he was fit, fit, fit. Now, several years after leaving the military he is a civilian who still works in the field of security, safety, teaching weaponry, and other top secret military stuff that sounds interesting and highly stressful. However, these days he works from home (and his couch) a great deal. And thus, somehow 80 pounds just snuck up on him and he just knows it's bad for him on so many levels. From showing up in front of the troops looking like he'd never been fit in his life, to struggling with climbing stairs at home (bad knee), he just decided it was time. To his favor, he and his girlfriend live a half a block from the beach in South Carolina, and have beach-walking as a cheap and easy exercise right at their doorstep. However, he also has every fried, cole-slawed, fat-oozing food joint around him wherever he looks! He's had a wake-up call that it's time to do something about it. Like Carol, he'd signed up for a month.

Jim, 57, is the guy I rode in the van with from the airport. He's a busy housing contractor in Indianapolis. He's got five kids and a bunch of grandkids and 40 pounds to lose. He also mentioned how tough it was just going up and down stairs. He says he's "Sick and tired of feeling sick and tired!"

But the real impetus that got him to the ranch is that one of his daughters is due to be married in May and he's latched

 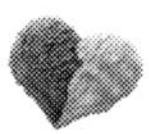

on to that as his goal – to be a great looking dad walking his daughter down the aisle. (Where had I heard that line before?)

One of his other issues was that he'd been on blood pressure and cholesterol meds for a long time, which he really hated. ("Have you read the side effects of those things?" he asked, his eyes looking panicked when he talked of it.) He was planning on weaning himself off them while he was there – with the blessing of his doc, if all went well. He was the type of guy that would do whatever Michael told him to do and would give it 100 percent. He was also the guy who would help anyone who needed something, although he enjoyed his alone time after the day was done and wasn't much of a social butterfly. His stint here – two weeks. Just like me.

Deb, or "Lil Deb," as Michael called her, was 52, and had already been at the ranch for six weeks, but still had 30 or so pounds to lose. She told me that she'd come here not just to lose weight, but to find some life answers. She'd quit her job, given her furniture to her daughter, and had come here looking for answers as to what she should do next in life. She was only with us for a few days as she'd been putting out feelers for a new job and after a couple of phone interviews, had to cut her stay early to go back to reality. She did tell me, however, that she'd found her direction at the ranch, far from the madding crowd. I'm not sure what it was but it's not important that I did. Only important that she did.

However, in her short time with us, Deb shared a positive vibe with us all. She even passed around a couple of photos of herself back when she had been a competitive body builder – eating 1,200 calories and working out a minimum of four hours per day to be in competing shape! Yikes! She shook her head telling us the story, as in, "Crazy, right?" We all had to admit, however, that her body-building photos were amazing. Can you say Ms. Atlas?

Since she wasn't with us long, I'll give you a quick-fast-forward of her stats upon leaving the ranch: Wt. loss: 20 pounds. Inches lost: 27. Attitude – amazing.

Lastly is our young pup, Todd. Every group has a Todd. Deb gave us the inside scoop about him since she'd been here with him the longest. He was 25. A college kid. Rich party boy. Forty pounds overweight. He was here for his 4th time in two years.

Did he lose weight each time? Yep, some. But being a typical youngster, Todd thought he had all the answers to everything, including weight loss. He loved to tell us that he could eat whatever he wanted as he'd burn it all off at the gym, for as hard as he worked out, which was nearly true. In fact, when he worked out he made the rest of us look like we were standing still. But then, that was part of his macho image. He'd drone on and on about when he went home how he was going to set up a workout regimen of his own, striving for 2-1/2 pounds per week instead of following Michael's plans for us.

For the amount of money this program cost (and for most of us that was hard-earned money) we all wondered if his parents had any idea how he was about as serious about the program as a drunken fraternity brother the night before finals.

I really wasn't sure why he kept coming back since he seemed to believe in exactly the opposite of whatever Michael had to teach us. But I guess he got *something* out of it. Ah, the young. By the end of our time there, he would at least prove to be entertaining in ways we didn't expect.

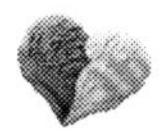

By the time Michael had wrapped up his welcome show, Todd hadn't shown up yet, but that apparently was his usual behavior. He'd been through orientation three times already and figured he'd get to know the newbies once everyone got settled in. No one waited for him.

And so, with everyone accounted for, and introductions done, Michael announced, "So I'm going to meet with each of you briefly, one-on-one, so that we can talk about your goals, your histories, any limitations ... that kind of thing. Of course, then you can ask me any questions you might have as well."

We all looked at each other and were likely too trembly in our boots to even know where to start at that point. We didn't know what we didn't know, as they say, and so we waited for more from Michael. It came quickly ...

"By the way" he announced, "your first test will come after dinner, so be sure to dress to work out. And don't stuff yourself. You're not going to want a full tummy for this."

We all looked at each other with a bit worried.

Was it too late to escape?

***

Michael called me in to his office first where he did a brief assessment of the basics: Height. 5'8'. Weight: 170.5 Numerous body measurements, some in places I never knew anyone ever measured!

"So, Mary Jo ... or do you prefer MJ?" he queried after he'd filled in all the basic boxes on my admission form.

"Either works," I smiled back. "Just not 'Mary.' Long story," I replied.

He glanced back at the form that detailed my medical history. I handed him another form from my doc at home.

"I brought a note from my doctor letting you know that there are no restrictions on me, per se. That, essentially, if something hurts or just doesn't feel safe for me to do it, then I shouldn't do it." I'd become pretty experienced with that situation over the years. He nodded as he glanced over my medical history.

"Wow," he studied me again. "You don't look like what I'd expect from someone with so much stuff." I suddenly felt my heart start racing as I formulated an answer to his question. These types of situations always leave me at a bit of a loss and somewhat pissed off. I was preparing some smart remark when he asked, "So what's your secret? You look great!"

I let out a deep breath and felt like the first hurdle had been jumped. It didn't look like he was going to judge me, rather, just needed to know what he could do to make my stay great. "Thanks," I replied, a bit unsure of what to do with his compliment. "I do try to fight it every step of the way ... my body gradually falling apart, that is. I just never thought it would happen so soon."

"Aw, you're far from falling apart. And you look ten years younger than you've a right to." He gave me one of his enticing smiles and went on. " You should see some of the folks who come here. And even more, you should see how different many of them are (in a good way) when they leave. And a lot of them have even more issues than you.

"The important thing for me," he went on, "is to know if there is anything specific you need from me or I need to know." His deep brown eyes were genuine and sincere. Yep. I knew I could trust this guy.

 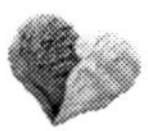

I thought for a moment. “You don’t have to worry about me leaving the crowd in the dust on any outing, but I won’t be the last either. Fortunately I have kept up a moderate gym attendance back in the real world, so I’m not like a complete newbie.

“I can’t kneel, so I’ll have to do some alternative moves from time to time. No knee pushups for me. And I’m a bit slow at getting up, so if you want to keep things moving along, you may want to offer me your hand instead of waiting for me to make it upright sooner or later.”

I thought for a minute. “Yep, I guess that’s about it.”

“No sweat. Piece of cake.” He jotted a couple more notes. “Now, with all the basics covered, Miss MJ, what really brought you here today?”

I thought about telling him how, at this point, *he* was the reason that brought me here. That the pure joy of admiring his Adonis body for two weeks would be plenty for me, but I behaved myself and shared with him my three goals: Shed a few pounds, get a big kick in the butt to get me off dead center, and practice some sense of a routine that could possibly help me improve on that skill at home.

And the biggest goal, which I didn’t tell him about, mostly because I hadn’t yet figured it out myself, was that I wanted to find my Miss Mojo again. With all that had happened to me in the last few years, she just seemed to have wandered off. Could I find her here? I prayed so. Could he be the one to help me find her? I hoped so.

***

By 7 p.m. the heat hadn't let up yet, the temp still hovering around 97 with about 80% humidity. But as directed, we all showed up in the parking lot after dinner, in our workout clothes, awaiting our fate. Deb had respectfully withdrawn. She'd done this activity a few times before and decided to sit this one out. But Todd, on the other hand, was chomping at the bit, ready to show off to the new arrivals. He seemed to gloat that he knew what was coming and no one else did. I guess it made him feel like some kind of expert or something. He jumped into the ranch's jeep, yelling to Michael, "Let's get this show on the road."

Michael directed us all to pile into the jeep as well as he slid into the driver's seat, started the engine, and drove us to the end of the mile-long lane up to the mailboxes that stood as lonely sentinels on the very empty country road.

As he did a U-turn and aligned the jeep facing back towards the ranch he said, "First of all, for those of you who can't live without your cell phones, you might want to know that this is the only place where you can get any reception whatsoever."

A huge groan floated on the air as we all started visualizing what that truly meant. Phone withdrawal, at the very least.

"Secondly, this is one of the best measurements of improvement you'll make here at the ranch. We call it, 'The Mile,' because it's exactly one mile from here to the bend in the driveway back near the mess hall. You are welcome to walk/run/crawl or whatever way you want to move yourselves along that gravel road. Then, at the end of your stay here, you'll run it again and do a comparison of the two."

"Damn right," shouted Todd. He was jumping and prancing like a prize fighter in the ring, ready to face his enemy. "I want to see just how much faster I can run it this time." He continued

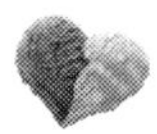

his boxer's jump, then added a few jabs and punches in the air to add to the impact.

"OK, everybody ready?" Michael scanned our faces, seeing the same expressions I am sure he always saw every time he sent folks out for this first task. Fear. Anguish. Anger. Terror. Shock. And any combination of the above. This was the activity that separated the men from the boys, so to speak, no gender slamming intended. It was the moment of truth that was the reason Cheryl kept from billing the credit cards until morning. If they couldn't handle this, simple walking for a mile, not to mention in the 90-something degree heat at 7PM – then they weren't going to make it for two weeks, especially in the full heat of the day. It was just that simple.

I realized that the MJ inside of me – the one who still had a few grains of Mojo left – was already sizing up my competition.

What to do? What to do? I was still debating what strategy I should take when suddenly Michael said, "Ready, set, go," as he set his stop watch and the games began. For a few moments no one really realized that things had begun but it only took that long for Todd to turn into a crazy nut and he blasted down the road ahead of us, assured of his success to come. He disappeared in a matter of moments.

The rest of us headed down the gravel road with whatever energy we could conjure up. I wondered just how much different this was going to be after two weeks of working our butts off, but for now, the job at hand was about all I could deal with.

We all took off a bit tentatively. But that seemingly short mile seemed more like twenty in a matter of moments. Especially since it was still so frickin' hot as hell at 7 p.m.

As everyone seemed to find their pace I realized that Jim and I were matching stride for stride at a very brisk walk, huffing and puffing as we traversed the ups and downs of the gravel road. The once-competitive track girl that I was back in high school was struggling with the decades-older me who was saying, "Don't be stupid. This is your first day, for God's sake. Don't kill yourself." Especially when I contemplated fully jogging this short distance and weighing that against my knee surgeon who isn't too keen on his patients jogging after knee replacements. I defaulted to the fast walk, going as fast as I could while always keeping one foot on the ground.

I felt Jim's presence and was determined to at least finish the race alongside him, if I could. I was completely tuned in to both my breathing and his huffing and puffing. I knew I had one advantage over him; he was a smoker of many years. I could hear it in his raspy breath.

Smoker or otherwise, he was pushing me – quite unaware he was doing so. And apparently, as he told me later – I was pushing him just as much. No words were spoken. This required serious concentration.

Chris had apparently thought that his intense training during many years of military service would bail him out during this seemingly simple mission. You know – falling back on experience kind of theory. He was certain that he could jog the whole thing, no problem. But he was in for quite a shock. He had leapt over the starting line with a fair amount of zest when Michael started us and appeared to be heading off to catch Todd.

Jim and I, in our deep concentration, hadn't given him a thought since he'd blasted ahead of us at the starting line and we were quite surprised when about 2/3 of the way through

 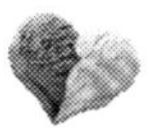

we saw him just barely ahead of us, all hunched over, still attempting to jog but barely making steps that look like walking. Besides just the cardio side of things, his knee was apparently killing him. He had a noticeable limp and was rubbing it, apparently to no avail.

Somehow before he'd actually begun the competition he must have thought that he could do so despite the fact that he'd not even been able to jog up his own flight of stairs back home in over five years! It's amazing how our brains lead us to make some stupid decision sometimes. Chris looked miserable as we caught up to him, showing no indication that he had enough energy to get a second wind, but finally stopped in his tracks, bent over at the waist, gulping in as much air as he could get.

I slowed down and offered him help (not exactly sure what that might have been), but he just waved me on and mouthed, "Go get 'em," without producing any sound. Jim looked a little uncertain about what to do as well, looking back from Chris to me and back. But there was really nothing any of us could do. Chris just had to catch his breath and quit pounding his knee. He needed ice, fluids, and to put his leg up. He really needed to wait for Michael to bring the jeep back for him. We could at least do that once we hit the finish line.

As I watched the whole scene unfold it occurred to me that all of this had happened in the short ten minutes that we'd been on this lonely, gravel road in the middle of nowhere, on the first challenge of our first day as boot campers. Oh, boy. This could be an interesting two weeks!

Suddenly I sensed an opportunity for me to edge up. With Chris out of the picture, it was only Jim and me, still neck and neck. (Not taking Todd into the equation at all – he was obviously in a league of his own.) But Jim and I were both hearing the competitive voices inside us, and without saying another word we fell back into our rhythm at the pace we were at before – possibly just a tad faster, yet neither of us switching up to a jog. (I wondered if he had bad knees too, but didn't have the breath to ask him.) I never knew I could walk as fast as I did then and there.

I found myself breathing in unison with Jim. Deep breath in, deep breath out. Steady. Determined. Pushing myself just a little more and a little more with each stride. It was all I could do to keep up with him. His pace pushed me. Thank God. I know I wouldn't have dug in as much as I did without him. And I don't think he wanted to be upstaged by a woman! So he pushed back as well.

All the time that the guys and I were struggling to get the lead, Carol brought up the rear, way, way behind us. Regrettably she was walking on her own without the advantage of a partner, which made everything that much harder. But onward she went, one step after the other. Almost as if she were marching. Swinging her water bottle in one hand and her other arm making big swings with each step. She told me later that this was the first time she'd pushed herself to her max in years. At the starting line she was convinced that she wouldn't make it and was terrified that she would somehow let us down. Instead, she met the challenge with stick-to-it-iv-ness and without complaint. I was only sad that I wouldn't be here to see her re-test at the end of her four weeks, since I'd be gone after only two. I'd bet money she'd make some serious improvements.

Back to the battle that was going on between Jim and me, things were definitely a'brewin. The end was in sight – only about a hundred yards to go. Michael, Todd, and Lil Deb were

 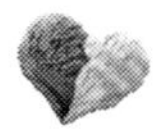

all jumping up and down, cheerleading for us at the finish line. I had managed to move slightly ahead of Jim but dared not turn around to look and see if I was right. Odds were likely I'd end up tripping on a piece of gravel or something and couldn't afford that now.

At last, with only about 25 yards to go, I decided I could pull out my secret weapons – my titanium knees – and see what stuff they had, making them insist that we wouldn't be telling my knee surgeon about any of this, so help me God.

I could feel the tension escalate between us and I could sense that he was running in maximum overdrive. I dug in my toes and pushed myself the last 20 yards to manage to come in ahead of him by 5 seconds!

I was pleased. A mile in 14:45 seconds. So glad I'd been a regular gym rat at home or I would have never pulled that off.

Suddenly, Carol appeared a couple of hundred yards away from the finish line, still trudging along and marching to her own drummer, and Todd sprung into action, running back down the drive until he met up with her. She looked exhausted but so pleased at the gesture, and her smile returned once again. She didn't even want to know her time. It didn't matter – she'd finished.

What inspired Todd, narcissistic pain-in-the-ass guy that he was, to support Carol like he did, none of us ever knew. But it wouldn't be the last time he surprised us all. It's just too bad that his opposite behaviors – more often like a jerk than a human being – were those that folks saw and would remember the most.

As for Chris, he limped painfully in, having to wait for another chance. There would be plenty more to come. No sense killing himself the first night, I am sure he was thinking.

"The Mile" was the first of many challenges we'd face during our time here. And it would be the last test for us at the end of our journey as well. I wondered how I'd hold up over the tough two weeks ahead.

Thus began our adventure.

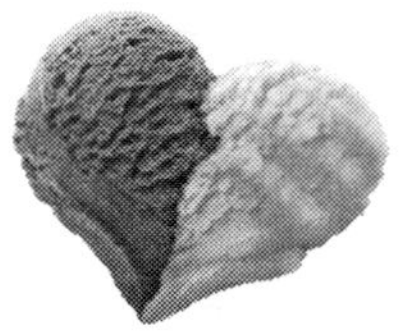

CHAPTER 21

Hello, My Body!

The sun rises early in this desert-like land, and it was streaming into the bunkhouse, waking me even before our alarms went off at 6:15. (We set both alarms in case we slept through one, as Michael had told us to be ready to rock and roll by 7 a.m.) Carol groaned, and burrowed down deeper in her nest, so I knew she was awake, but she didn't make any effort to move from her snugly cocoon. "Good morning, Bunkie," I said, my throat sounding scratchy. She just groaned again, indicating she just wasn't feeling like talking yet. Fair enough. I stopped nagging.

I could hear the horses nickering not far away, as it was their breakfast time and they were impatiently stomping and complaining that the cowboys throwing them hay and grain were taking much too long. Once fed, an eerie quiet settled in as they munched away, and the nickering turned to a rhythmic grinding that brought a peaceful feeling to the valley.

As I climbed out of my bunk, the first screaming muscles reminded me of last night's escapade. I made a bee line for my supplies and dumped four Advil in my hand, tossed them down with a little water that I had left in yesterday's water bottle, and prayed that they would work soon. My calves were definitely not happy. Not sure what other body parts might be complaining yet, since right now the calves were definitely number one. But one crisis at a time, I always say. I had to wonder how bad everyone else was feeling, especially Chris. Sure hope, for his sake, he iced his knee and pounded the Advil after torturing it during The Mile. I bet he was in no rush to get out of bed.

Just putting my contacts in that early seemed like torture. But I mastered that chore and managed to get myself dressed and headed to the lounge (our headquarters) while Carol, moving much slower than I, was about 15 minutes behind me.

We all slowly trickled in, each of us bringing in our own version of morning personality. Those addicted to coffee, hiding behind their steaming mugs; those who couldn't function without knowing what was going on in the outside world, glued to NBC news on TV. And those addicted to the Web were busy texting their folks back home about last night's torture, no doubt.

Just then Chris limped in wearing a black, neoprene knee brace, trying not to show that he was definitely in pain, but being ex-military, one pushes on. Hoo rah! as the Marines say! I hoped he knew what he was doing.

Deb, smiling and relaxed, knew full-well what the day had ahead for us and she could anticipate what was coming next. For her the day's activities were probably a pleasant challenge, and not the chore many of us were anticipating.

Michael was already there, chatting and joking with everyone, still dancing with the ants in his pants. I wondered if he had ADHD or too much coffee. Finally, everyone except Todd had arrived.

 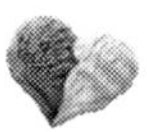

"Good morning," Michael started. "How are we all feeling this morning?" A giant groan leaked from most everyone. You'd think we were all hungover or something. Needless to say, Michael had seen this reaction many Monday mornings before our crowd had been the guinea pigs for the day, and he refused to let us wallow in our misery. We were here to grab success, after all! His high energy had already begun to create a positive charge that seemed to get everyone re-focused in a good way.

He looked at Chris. "You doing OK, man?" (I smiled to myself – they had to exchange their macho thing.)

Chris nodded, with a bit of a grimace and gave Michael a look that said, "Don't single me out. Everyone here is hurting! I'm not special."

Taking Chris at his word, Michael moved on to the day's tasks and passed out a printed agenda of week one's workouts. We all tried to contain ourselves as we examined what looked to be impossible. Everyone's eyes grew bigger by the minute, as the realization of what we were in for was just hitting home for some. As if last night's demonstration wasn't enough.

"We're going to start every morning with a Wake Up Warm Up at 7 before breakfast to get your blood pumping. That could be a quick hike around the ranch like today, a brief fitness testing, or some well-needed stretching, like I bet many of you could use today."

"WHAT?" I thought. "A workout before we even eat? Are you kidding me?"

"Then we'll have breakfast at 8," he continued. "From 8:30 to 10 today we'll do some assessments in the gym, where I will get a handle on your stamina and skill level. Then, there's a snack from 10 to10:30. From 10:30 until noon we're going to do some cardio, followed by lunch from 12 to 1."

I looked around and wondered just how everyone was going to manage such a feat, myself included. And this was just the beginning. I had thought I was doing pretty well back home doing some kind of cardio three days a week. But that was going to look like nothing compared to what this schedule was looking like.

Michael went on ..."The afternoon starts at one; we might do something like Tabata, which is a new breed of workout where you work super high intensity for 20 seconds, then rest for 10 seconds, and keep repeating for a total of 4 minutes per exercise. Believe me, it's sounds easy, but it's not. But research is showing that it can be as effective as a full 45 minute workout. So for any of you who simply don't have the time to fit a workout into your busy day, you might really like this one."

We were all growing increasingly concerned, so he stepped up the positive info a bit.

"At three there will be one more afternoon snack followed by water aerobics, taught by my colleague, Katie, which is not only a calorie burner but it's a hell of a lot of fun as well – especially if you like water basketball. Then, wind down at the end of the day and let yourself relax in the cooling waters of the indoor pool."

The word *relax* got our attention! Then he ended his speech with a couple more quick highlights ...

"Other fun activities we'll be doing while you're here include yoga, Zumba, relaxation, nutrition, hypnosis, an obstacle course, and a few others. I will even be cooking for you one night, demonstrating my chef skills as I clue you in to what healthy food looks and tastes like."

 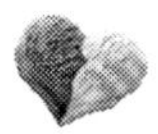

“Stop flapping your lips, Michael, we’re burning daylight,” Deb piped up from the chair in the corner. She stood up and headed for the door and the energy shifted once again. We all felt a twinge of excitement returning. Her success was the best advertisement we could have had.

Michael looked at our improving expressions and said, “What she said. Let’s go!” And we took the first steps into what was still a big unknown.

***

I never found out just how big the ranch was but I guessed it was several hundred acres. The trails were well worn, since they’re mostly used by the city slickers on the dude ranch side of thing, for trail riding a couple times per day. Other than our having to dodge horse manure, the trails were mostly not too difficult to traverse, although they were by no means flat. The up and down nature of the land had us huffing and puffing one minute and catching our breath on the downhill side the next. And occasionally, there were some spots that were purely loose gravel, which, if not navigated well, could leave one slip-sliding away down the hillside.

I’d found a pair of hiking poles in the lounge and figured my knees would appreciate any support they could get. And did that prove to be smart! I would end up using them on every hike we took, both to assist in balance and in climbing in and around some mighty huge rocks along the way that we faced on every hike.

The barren land that I had watched on the drive out here was a lot more intimate from this angle. Everywhere were beautiful prickly pear cacti with their bright yellow blossoms attracting not only us to their beauty, but all the bees and insects that lived off their produce as well. (Note to oneself, however: mind your step. This could be really ugly if you fall into those spines!)

By now, we had settled in to a grouping that would pretty much remain unchanged over the two weeks we'd be together. Of course Todd was always at the front, running for several yards then plopping himself on a big rock, then waiting for the rest of us to catch up by spreading his shirtless body full-out on the rock to work on his tan. Then he'd run headlong again and repeat the pattern, of course looking like he'd run a marathon with his exertion, sweat pouring off of him in a matter of minutes. He seemed to like wearing sweat like an Olympic medal.

Chris and Jim followed Todd, although without all the Superman behavior. Their theory was more like: We're tough. We're strong. We're guys. (Although after last night's events I figured they were actually holding back a little for the time being, doing their best not to have a repeat any time soon.) The three chatted non-stop while Carol and I were mostly using our lungs just to breathe in that hot, humid air.

Carol, Lil Deb and I took up the rear, our theory being more like "slow and steady wins the race." We kept our chatting to a minimum, although Lil Deb, who'd had six weeks to adjust to the climate and the work, didn't seem the worse for the wear and carried most of the conversations as we three gals brought up the rear. Michael, the roadrunner, jumped back and forth, making sure everyone was doing alright ... especially us stragglers.

 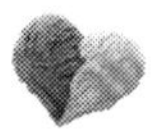

"How's it going, ladies?" he'd inquire periodically as he would fall back into step with us, despite our slower pace, us being the weakest links. Then he'd grab his cell phone, set it to video, and film us slowly maneuvering the terrain. "Smile, everybody," he grinned and narrated his filmmaking, "Yes, ladies and gentlemen, we're here today at Rancho Cortez with Carol, MJ, and Lil Deb as they climb the dusty trail in the beautiful Hill Country of Texas. Give us a thumb's up, ladies," and he zoomed in on each of us, giving us no rest until he got a thumb's up and a big smile from each of us.

"Thank you for documenting this, Michael," Deb replied; her obvious positive energy such a welcome glimmer in a world that's so negative all the time. It became obvious to anyone who spent any time with her that she'd definitely found her direction at Rancho Cortez and couldn't wait to put it to some positive use shortly. I was sad not to get to spend two weeks with her, since she was apparently leaving in a matter of days. I think I could have learned a thing or two from Deb.

It was an awesome start to the day. I think everyone was doing better, once we were actually rolling along and doing something fun, at the same time burning calories. The vistas we looked back on from the top of one of the Hill Country's hills was spectacular. We could see for miles and took tons of photos for posterity.

While it had only been about 30 minutes since our hike had begun, the effort we were putting in, the heat and humidity creeping up on us, and the fact that most of us hadn't eaten since 6 p.m. last night, left us starving. We wrapped up the photo-taking and headed back to breakfast, pleased with this morning's outing after all, and perhaps just a little less terrified of what was to come.

Just then, and despite being in the slow group, Deb misstepped in the loose gravel, her feet went out from under her, and she went sliding down the hillside for several feet before coming to a halt against a big rock. The sound of sliding gravel made us all catch our breath, not exactly sure for a moment just what had transpired and if, God forbid, anyone was hurt. We all hurried to where she lay and were glad to see that while she was a little lumped and bumped, she'd not hurt anything badly, although I suspect that under her torn shorts, where the worst of the damage had been done, would likely resemble a bad case of road rash with accompanying nasty bruising. That was gonna sting for a bit. And be pretty ugly longer than that.

"You sure you're OK?" I asked, the nurse in me from years ago taking over the scene as I assessed the situation, brushing the layer of sand off Deb's face as she picked herself up.

"It's nothing," she reassured all of us, as she tried to get the sand out of her hair. "I'll be fine. Thanks, everyone, but really, I'll be OK." She limped around a bit, getting re-situated, and I knew she'd been hurt more than she was letting on, but not so bad to need a trip to the ER. Unfortunately, she still had to make it back on a sore body. And needed to be packed in ice as soon as possible.

The positive energy of earlier had slowly dissipated but Lil Deb pasted on one of her best smiles and started down the trail as if she could walk the exact same way she had climbed up the hill. Nice idea, but she learned pretty quickly that wasn't going to be the case and begrudgingly let Jim and Chris support her on each side, being especially cautious to avoid any further loose gravel.

 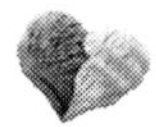

Well, we all made it back without further crisis and got Deb set up in her room. She'd smartly chosen a private room for her time at the ranch, so wasn't in the low rent district that Carol and I shared. She'd certainly be more comfortable that way. She even had her own TV, another thing missing from the rustic bunkhouse. We left her with her ice pack, a to-go plate of breakfast that someone had brought for her, and her TV remote so she wouldn't have to get up for awhile. And strict orders to lay low for the rest of the day. And believe it or not, she didn't fight the orders.

And the next day she was back for more.

One tough cookie.

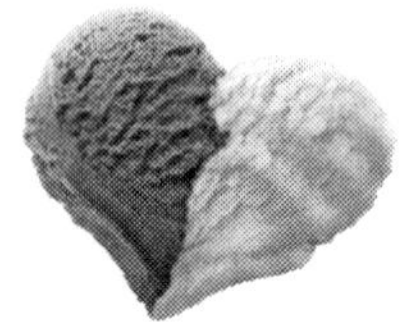

CHAPTER 22

The Rest Of Day One

By the time our early morning jaunt had come to an end we were starving and headed to the mess hall as quickly as our tired legs could carry us.

The mess hall was a bit unusual in that it was the one area where dudes and boot campers alike were in the same place at the same time. And while it all looked the same to an outsider, we boot campers knew better.

Why?

Well, for starters, the food was simple and there was only one entree choice per meal; this was not an order-off-the-menu kinda place! And the nearest McDonalds was a good 30 minutes away by car. So what you saw was what you got. And the cooks doled out the servings. No waste there. You could always go back for seconds if you wanted to. They didn't mind, but they were sure not gonna be wasteful either.

But the big thing was that the dudes certainly didn't come to the ranch to eat diet food and boot campers didn't come to camp thinking that temptation would be so close by.

Let me explain; the cooks made two meals at each mealtime. They prepared healthy, low calorie, low fat options for

 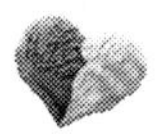

the boot campers, and of course always a giant salad and fruit bar that both types of guests were welcome to partake in. But for the dudes and dudettes, they also offered more typical Texas fare like BBQ, hot dogs, cheese burgers, biscuits and gravy, waffles, pancakes, and worst of all, they made incredible brownies, pies, and chocolate chip cookies that got your tongue a-drooling.

BUT, if a boot camper wasn't happy with the light version of a meal, and decided to indulge with the dudes in the higher caloric version of said meal, no one was going to slap his or her hand and say, "No, no, no. This is NOT your food." Or if you desperately wanted one of those amazing cookies no one would clobber you with a ruler like the nuns back in grade school or call you bad or evil. The thought was, we were all grownups. The choice was up to us. (What a concept.)

After all, by the time we went home, there were not going to be any food police there, arresting us for unhealthy eating, were there? No cook to choose the boring lite food to put on your tray because she knows the reason you're here is to quit putting the bad food in your mouth. And none of your boot camp buddies would be there to give you "The Look" when you actually did take something from the dude food.

"The Look," was an expression some of us used when we checked out what sinful stuff our buddies were eatin' and we wanted to eat the not-so-healthy things that they chose *just as much as they did*, but we were able to keep the jealous side of our minds in check. At least for that moment in time. "The Look" actually translated to, "God, I wish I had the guts to eat that stuff too; I want it desperately. *But*, I'm really a groupie and wouldn't dare take such a monumental step as being seen eating the bad stuff with everyone watching. So instead, I'll give you the look and you'll know exactly how pissed off I feel about the whole, rotten thing." Then you'll go off to eat your delectable and the Looker will turn away, knowing that the message had been delivered and life could go on. No judging. Just communicating.

I do have to admit to swiping a few of those evil cookies myself a few times. (Which I'm convinced that they left out on the kitchen counter after lunch, fiendishly, just tempting us with their unhealthy, but oh so delectable sugar and chocolate.) I really didn't believe that, but surely wanted to.

That morning, however, I think we would have all eaten three day-old, left-over pizzas, we were so hungry. Instead the cooks had made us scrambled eggs, chicken, and pulled pork. Who could complain? It hit my tongue and exploded with flavor, causing me to salivate like a lion over his kill and breathe slowly and deeply to make the scent of it last. I truthfully couldn't remember having such a warm, satisfying, glorious meal as that breakfast in a long, long time.

I don't think any of us spoke for at least ten minutes while we inhaled the wondrous but simple meal. We definitely got our necessary protein intake. While we were nearly having an intimate experience with the food, none of us even noticed that the dudes were guzzling down French toast, as well as biscuits and gravy while we were inhaling boring protein. Yet, for that one particular meal anyway, we thought we were luckier than the wanna-be cowboys ever would be.

***

 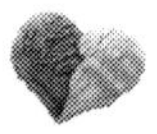

It was hard to believe how much had happened already and it was only about 9 a.m. – time for the next round of exercise. With Lil Deb tucked away for the day and our tummies full of pulled pork and more, we finally had the right attitude to take the next step.

The indoor gym was a couple of hundred yards from the lounge, up a bit of an incline requiring that we all bend forward slightly, digging in with our toes, calling upon a little bit of energy and strength we'd found on the hike this morning to get us up the hill. With only minor huffing and puffing this time, we all arrived in one piece.

The gym was bright, roomy, and typical in every way but one ... it had almost no machines. I saw one rower but that was it. But everything else we'd ever need was there: dumb bells, kettle bells, weight benches, mats, heavy ropes, Bosu® balls, and everything in between. And thank God it was air conditioned as the external temp was already registering in the 90's. They reminded me that it was a dry heat, but who are they kidding? Mid-90's is mid-90s: HOT, especially when you're working out as we would continue to be reminded over the days just walking from building to building, not to mention the upcoming promised hikes!

When we wandered in, Michael was already there with his music playing LOUDLY, as he danced and swayed to the tunes. There indeed was a huge mirror, as I knew there would be. You gotta have your priorities straight, right? We all chose our spots on the floor, which we pretty much clung to for the rest of our stay, and jumped into Michael's schedule.

First, he put us through some serious stretching since we hadn't really done any before the hike. I heard things creaking and groaning, and the sounds didn't all come from just my body either. (They did say there was a Jacuzzi® here for later, right? Plus a small outdoor pool and a small indoor one where we were going to have water aerobics at some point. The temperature in at least one of those bodies of water should feel good for soaking at the end of the day.) That was my goal – just make it to the Jacuzzi in one piece.

Next, more testing to see what we had to give. Like how many sit-ups could we do in one minute? Or how many push ups … that kind of thing. Just more "before" information to have as evidence of our improvements when we left.

By the time 3 p.m. had rolled around we'd had 2 morning workouts, a snack, lunch, and one of our afternoon workouts. We had snack and a break until 3. Most of us chugged the chocolate protein shakes then raced back to our bunks to get some shut eye. We all were beat and weren't done yet for the day.

But this time we had something a little less punishing to look forward to after break – water aerobics in the coolness of the indoor pool! So an hour later we returned rested and ready to get into our swim suits, with most of the newbies having no idea what water aerobics was about.

Our instructor, Katie, a lovely young lady around 21 or so, was the daughter of the ranch owners. She was a highly skilled horse woman as her first love, and was busy with the dude program most of the time. In that job she was clad in skinny Levi's that hugged her curves as if they were painted on, an equally snug-fitting ranch type shirt with the pearl snap buttons, her dusty cowboy boots, of course, the big silver trophy belt buckle that indicated that she's won some competition or other, and

 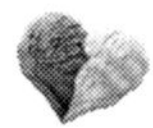

of course her straw cowboy hat strategically perched on her long, brunette curly locks. She was on the shy side but helpful nonetheless.

At least, that's how she appeared when she was in the mess hall or whenever she was around the dudes and dudettes. But how she came clothed to teach water aerobics that first day – in a very tiny bikini that embraced her perfect body and all its curves – was as an eye-opening, head-turning, jaw-dropping, stop-men-in-their-tracks-looking nymph instead of what most of us expected: some lifeguard-looking middle-aged chick who taught CPR for a living.

I suddenly realized that she must be to the guys what Michael was to the women guests: eye candy and entertainment. Fair is fair, after all. Although I don't think that Katie had a clue that she was absolutely stunning and it was probably a good thing that we were all in about four or more feet of water – waist high – as the boys all ogled her with their eyes in between following her instructions as to how to do the exercises in the water.

There would likely be talk later that night of some other things that "came up" during water aerobics! Just a few extra benefits for the poor guys too exhausted to do anything at the end of the day, even if they'd had a gun put to their heads! Ah well, this was only Day 1. The future was yet unwritten.

Now don't get me wrong – she was a young, naive gal, sweet as all get-out and a bit new to teaching anyone anything, but very eager to try and very willing to take suggestions on how she could make the class better. I believe she was in college taking courses in human kinesiology or something, so she obviously was smart as well. Bottom line: she provided entertainment for the guys as they learned to exercise in the water, and we women could just keep looking at her out of the corner of our eyes, sizing her up in our own ways, wishing we would have ever looked like her even once in our lives.

And so, once Katie got the initial excitement (no pun intended) under control, she showed us how to exercise in waist-deep water while she performed the movements on the pool edge so we could better see everything from above. Thirty squats followed by 30 leg kicks followed by 30 arm reaches over our heads, followed by 30 more of these and 30 more of those … she kept us working from one movement to the next; chop-chop.

Then, after a refreshing workout, Katie introduced us to pool basketball where we split into teams and had to throw basketballs to the opposite side of the pool through the ceiling rafter until we were exhausted. When we stopped, we realized that we'd actually been having fun! And Carol had been the high scorer for the day, even beating out the guys! Topping the day off on a much higher note than where it had begun. We all thanked Katie profusely, to which she beamed with happiness, knowing she'd done a good job. And we left the pool starving once again but filled with a great sense of completion.

I headed to the small outdoor pool after that, by myself, while everyone else headed to their rooms for whatever they needed to do before dinner. I just needed some time to regroup and think about everything and see if I couldn't catch a few late afternoon rays on my pasty, white body.

The constant hum of all the air conditioning units became part of the ranch sounds, and after awhile I didn't even hear

 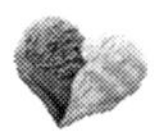

them. I also realized that I heard country music floating across the compound with the radio DJ crooning in his lilting voice through a camouflaged speaker that looked like it was just one of the rocks in the terrain. Yep, where else but in Texas?

By the time I'd spent 20 minutes grilling each side of myself, it was time to get ready for dinner. So I headed back to the Bunk House Hotel where surprisingly enough I found Carol showered, dressed, and heading to the lounge to check emails before dinner. Apparently it was about the only place you could get any sort of Wi-Fi and if anyone could get it to work, it would be Carol.

"What a day," I muttered as I stripped out of my still-wet bathing suit as Carol grabbed her laptop and headed for the door.

"Yep, but it was fun, too, wasn't it?" Even her eyes were smiling. It was good to see her happy at the end of this long day. "By the way, Deb is fine. I checked on her after we were done and not only was she up and around, she got a call from a possible employer and has a phone interview with some company tomorrow.

"Wow, looks like it turned out to be a good day for all," I said, smiling back. Indeed it had been a day with much to learn and absorb. Speaking of which, I remembered to pull out my laptop for later when we got back, as I wanted to make some notes about everything that had happened today and every day I was there, cuz you never know, I might write a book about it or something!

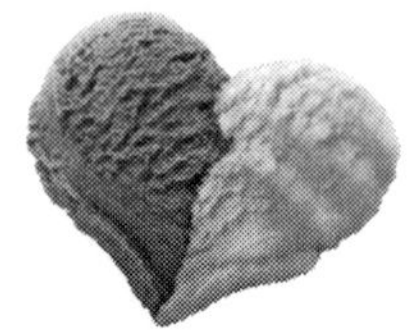

CHAPTER 23

Falling Stars

You could tell that everyone was starving as we circled the mess hall awaiting the sound of the dinner bell that would allow us to enter the cozy space we shared with the dudes and dudettes and any munchkin dudes, three times per day. I couldn't help thinking how funny it was how we might as well have been in 1960's Alabama; there was an undercurrent of discrimination that had nothing to do with the color of our skin but rather, whether we were the ones here on a vacation, spending money lavishly on fancy rooms or relaxing strolls mounted upon a fancy steed, or if we were seen most of the time wearing soaking wet workout clothes, dripping sweat into our plates, or heard moaning and groaning should anyone pass the gym at the right time of day. There was no resentment or anything – more like neither side knew how to cross over to the other's camp and blend in. So we just stayed to our own corners.

One day two bus loads of Japanese teenagers and their chaperones came to do some filming of a cowboy in action. The owner, Larry Cortez, showed them some roping tricks and God knows what other cowboy things, which left them

 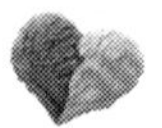

all fascinated. You should have seen the mess hall that night. Yikes. It was almost standing room only and most of them didn't speak English. At the end of the night they climbed back on the bus to head off for other American exotic vacation spots. We never knew who might show up tomorrow.

What made it especially hard was that the dude folk were typically short-term, I was to learn, like 1- 2 days. So it's easy to see how it was harder making new friends each night only to have them gone the next morning. And thus, our workout friendships and teamwork began to grow as we got to know each other more.

"Anyone want to join me on a walk to the mailboxes to use your phones?" I inquired as I stacked my dishes for the kid who cleaned up after mealtime. That got the ball rolling as everyone finally realized that we didn't have to be anywhere for once. Yet they were so tired they were afraid to even sit down for fear of dozing off and then missing their opportunity to call their loved ones from across the country who had likely been waiting to hear their voices all day.

Of course the idea of walking two more miles before bedtime made a couple folks stop and re-think the idea. They had forgotten 'til now that supposedly the only decent cell reception was up at the top of that damned gravel road leading to the mailboxes. Yep, a mile each way.

In my mind it was a perfect, relaxing night, finally. The temperature had dropped to something livable. The sun slowly sinking in the West had set the sky on fire, dabbing it with rich hues of red, orange, pink, and yellow. A painter's joy. That, combined with the overwhelming sounds of the cicadas buzzing away like a band of harmonica players trying to get in tune, set a different mood from the rest of the day for me. It spelled peace. I could already find something stirring in me, maybe not yet as powerfully as Deb had gone through, but I liked the uncertain feeling in the pit of my stomach. I realized that I was already glad I'd come.

Funny, I didn't even feel the strong pull to use the damned phone like everyone else was having a hissy about. I just felt the need to walk at my own pace and no one telling me how long I had to do so. And so, while the others debated, I headed down what I began to know as "my road," as you'll see over time.

Realizing I'd headed out all ready, Jim and Todd joined me, only hurried by the appetite and the pull of friends or family at home. Wisely, Chris declined and decided to ice his leg and watch TV. Yep, he was one of the smart ones with a private room, which had come in handy.

They were in a funny mood that evening. Probably pure exhaustion. Todd, of course, had to be the center of attention and as he was the expert on everything Rancho Cortez, this being his fourth trip. He started sharing stories of his experiences, including his many falls off the proverbial wagon on what he called his "Free Days," when he allowed himself to eat anything he wanted once a week.

I didn't want to listen to any more of his teenage bragging, which he should have lost years ago, and so I pretended to bend down to remove a rock from my shoe and let them move ahead.

It was funny walking behind them, Jim simply marching on like a soldier and Todd nearly dancing his way up the road. Ah, the energy of the young. I was happy just to wander slowly, enjoying all the tiny, purple flowers that lived in with the weeds, catching a glimpse of some cows or horses grazing behind the rusty barbed wire fence, or a lazy hawk floating overhead looking for some dinner. It was so far from my world and felt so safe. I said a little prayer thanking God for sending me to this place.By the time we got to the mailboxes we each opened up our phones to call someone at home we hoped was missing us, and that we likely were missing ourselves. I think Jim called his kids. Not sure who Todd called. And I called my daughter. I caught her as she was heading to the ER for some train wreck that was coming in but I had her attention for about five minutes.

"Hey, how's it going, Mom?" she asked, although I could tell she only had time for the short version.

"It's great, Honey. Hard, but great. So far, I'm really glad I've come." And so far, I was.

"Good for you, Mom." I knew she hadn't been really certain why I'd felt the need to make this trip, but she respected me and my decision to do so and just wanted me to be happy.

"But boy, it's hot here," I said as I wiped my sweating brow yet again. "The gym's air conditioned but they tell us we'll take some lengthy hikes while we're here and I'm doubting that the temps will drop just for us hikers."

"You'll do it, Mom. You're tough." That's what she always said about me ... that I'm the strongest, and sometimes the toughest woman she knew. I wasn't always sure that was a good thing but in this case it felt like a compliment and I was going to take it as such. Adding one of the first ingredients to my "Getting my Mojo back" plan.

I could tell she was rushed so told her I loved her and missed her and let her run to whatever pile of broken bones awaited her in the ER. Guess she had enough Mojo for her life's direction, at least at this point on her journey. She was passionate about orthopedic surgery and as her Mama, I couldn't have been more proud. You always wish as a mom that you give your kids what they need to make it in the big world and when you see those lessons come through in how they live their lives, it's one of the most rewarding moments of your life.

Just one more warm fuzzy to add to my already wonderful day.

I noticed that the sun was getting awfully damned low over the hillside and motioned to the boys that it would be dark soon. Then, I slowly started back down that gravel road again, as they wrapped up their calls behind me.

By the time we made it back it was nearly dark as the stars started twinkling through the stratosphere. We were so far out from civilization that the sky was perfect for watching for shooting stars ... no interfering lights from the city. It didn't take long, once full night was upon us, for the light show to begin and it was magnificent.

I returned to the outdoor pool area and pulled up a lounge chair, stretching out to watch the display, which sent out flying orbs every few minutes as I sat there open-mouthed, awed by the beauty of something I'd seen only a few times before in my life. It was like someone was magically painting the sky with random lines of white sparkles, sometimes with several overlapping at the same time; shooting left, shooting right, "stand up, sit down, fight, fight, fight," I thought, amused that the old cheer from high school was rolling out of my memory banks just then. I could barely look away, I was so hypnotized by the heavenly action and made sure I thanked God above for sharing His wonder with me yet again on this special day. The light show felt like it was a special gift just from Him to me.

In the background the dudes and their families were enjoying making s'mores and getting all their little fingers and faces sticky with chocolate and marshmallow paste. They were listening to cowboy Larry strumming his guitar and singing his favorite cowboy songs at a huge campfire in the center of their circle. It was snapping and popping and shooting red-hot embers up to several feet away, but the pit was big enough to handle even a good-sized crowd. I'd bet you that most of those kids had never even experienced a real bonfire before. I felt a little twinge of gratitude as I watched them enjoying the little things in life.

At last, I called it quits and headed to the bunk house to type up some thoughts and to put my aching body to bed. Tomorrow was only about six hours away.

Guess I'd better hurry.

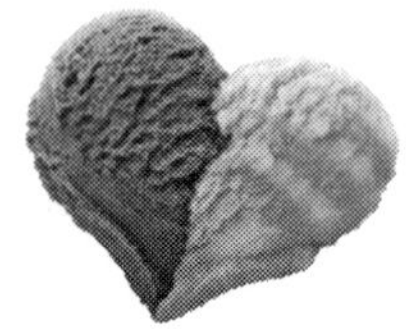

CHAPTER 24

Enchanted Rock

The days flew by. Each day still began with the Wake Up Workout before breakfast, whether it be a quick cardio stint, or another short hike around the property, or just a good stretch session to ease our aching muscles, for which most of us had been popping Advil or Tylenol around the clock to make it through the next activity while still paying the price for the last one.

By 8 a.m. the ringing of the mess hall bell got us salivating for breakfast, as we dug in to our usual meals of eggs, meat of some kind, fruit, oatmeal, and, oh yes, did I say eggs? I'd never eaten so many eggs in my life. I also would steal an apple and throw it in my backpack for a quick pick-me-up I would undoubtedly need sometime during the day, despite the two scheduled snacks.

We would have two morning workouts and two afternoon ones, unless it was a day that we went on a huge hike in one of the state parks and were away from the ranch too long to do the more structured activities. Not to worry; those hikes, unlike the short one at the property, kicked our butts like nothing else, so it wasn't that we were getting away with anything!

They did give us Sunday off completely, thank God. Although that first Sunday that Chris and Carol and I went into the closest little burg just to escape the ranch for a while, we fell off the wagon royally and ate real food for lunch – French fries and all! There were grins all around as we savored our fare as if we'd never eaten anything so decadent. Then gave ourselves credit for at least not buying dessert! Unlike Chris, Jim, and I, both Carol and Todd had their own cars, so in theory could go to town to pig-out or otherwise, anytime they'd a mind to. And while Carol pretty much stayed away from the evils of the small town and its sinful fruits, Todd paid frequent visits to town and other places unknown. In fact he usually headed down the gravel drive each evening after dinner and never shared much about his evening adventures with us. Ah, the young have so much energy!

The days were never boring. Michael had us moving from one activity to the next, from circuit training to ab work to free weights to Tabata to strength circuit to stretching, and more.

While it may have seemed that we were working out from morning to sunset every day, that wasn't exactly true. There were brief snack and rest times scheduled throughout the day, and boy, did we use them! Many of us learned to power nap! It was amazing how 30 minutes of sleep was enough to refresh us to come back for yet another workout, after barely finishing one that had us begging to quit just an hour earlier.

There were other activities as well. A couple of local experts stopped by to introduce us to Yoga, Zumba, relaxation, and self-hypnosis. A masseuse came in a couple of times per week and we kept him busy working out our knots.

A nutritionist gal showed us how to cook healthy and yet still make things that were good to eat and not difficult to prepare. And even Michael cooked for us a couple of nights, demonstrating that he had skills outside the gym.

Despite the fact that we were constantly exhausted, sleep was not easy. For me, a night owl under usual circumstances, I tried to tuck myself in around 10 p.m. but ended up waking at 5 a.m., unable to go back to sleep. The others were frustrated as well. No one was sleeping through the night. However, many were finding cat naps between workouts to be a mixed blessing. While it might have helped us get through the next workout, it may have also messed with our normal sleep patterns at night. Ugh.

A very sad day caught us all off-guard when we turned on the TV one morning to hear about Robin Williams' suicide. We were all in shock. How could someone who appeared so totally happy all the time, someone who had himself made millions of people around the world laugh themselves silly, find himself so sad as to take his own life? It was pretty quiet in the lounge that next 24 hours while the media kept trying to sort out the details of the situation. It was a sad day for the whole world.

***

One of my very favorite parts of my time at the ranch was our trip to hike Enchanted Rock in Llano County, a bit of a drive away but so worth it. Michael had tried to describe the enormity of the mountain but it was impossible to picture. In fact, once we were there it was even impossible to take any

 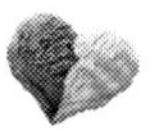

kind of picture of it that would even come close to representing it in its entirety. Not even a panorama camera did it justice.

Viewing it made you think that perhaps aliens had dropped a huge, pink, granite bowl upside down in the middle of nowhere, with a few dribs and drabs of whatever was in the bowl, splattering the landscape as well. Then all of it froze in place forever.

It was indeed a huge, pink, round granite mountain in the middle of nowhere, drawing visitors from all over the world. Some fun facts about the place: it covers 640 acres and the rock itself rises to an elevation of 1,825 feet above sea level and is considered a State Natural Area. Archaeologists believe people have been coming to the rock for over 12,000 years, something they learned from arrow heads and other tool remnants that could be dated via today's technology.

There were many Indian legends in the rock's history. Things like, if you spent the night on the mountain, you would become invisible. Beliefs that ancient tribes found it as a holy portal to other worlds. There is one story of a man who was eaten by the rock where he was exposed to various spirits for two days until the rock spit him out again. Also some legends had it that there were the sounds of a sobbing woman who had watched the slaughtering of her people there. Many tribes felt it had magical powers, thus the name.

We were all definitely impressed and Michael was eager to show us everything. Even Todd was excited to share one of his state's many wonders with us and filled us with stories and details as if he were our own personal tour guide. He was almost like a ten-year-old kid eager to teach his parents how to use his new X-Box he'd just gotten for Christmas, and his energy and passion came through loud and clear. Everything was still all about him being center stage, but at least for a few moments it was not about him being a jerk. There was a decent kid inside there somewhere.

From the entrance, the huge, pink boob of a rock looked enormous but with a gradual sloping from top to bottom from all sides. It certainly didn't look horribly steep or daunting. In fact, I had chatted on the phone with my brother in Texas the preceding night about the next day's activity and he shared with me how a 75-year-old relative had climbed the rock recently himself and without difficulty, even raving at the experience when he was finished. Surely, if he could do it, so could I? I'd done a lot of hiking on some pretty moderately difficult locations before – even after all the surgeries, but my lost Mojo was just making me question myself at every turn lately. At least, it seemed, whenever the tough got going.

As I took a look with the binoculars Michael had brought I saw quite a number of people on the top of the big, pink thing already. Obviously early morning hikers, since it was only 10:30 or so and they appeared to be heading back. It certainly didn't seem to be any biggie from *this* angle.

The trails leading to the rock itself were in great shape, consisting mostly of sand or else just more of the granite, which the entire rock was made of. There were also little markers of small, stacked rocks pointing hikers towards the best routes up the mountain, in case anyone feared losing their way. Not that anyone could get lost on the mountain itself – it had barely a scraggly remnant of a tree on it. Just a big naked boob with full sun all day overlooking a landscape below of that same sandy, hot, dried juniper tree vista.

 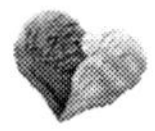

I squinted through my sunglasses at the cooking sun and remembered today's forecast: another sunny day in the 90's.

We made sure our water bottles were full and hit the trail, with the boys, as usual, taking off with a spurt to get the lead and Michael hanging back to make sure that Carol and I would be OK. Carol was hiking with one pole these days and I thanked my lucky stars that I had two or I was pretty darned sure that I would never make it up to the top. In fact, as Michael was jabbering with us about his many experiences at the place I was assessing just how steep the climb was going to be. And, honestly, if I'd be able to make it with my titanium knees I'd only had for three years and had not tested in such a situation before.

The granite itself was dry and edgy to walk on, not at all like the smooth-surfaced granite countertops at home in my kitchen. Although, they were also just flat enough and smooth enough that I wouldn't have wanted to be coming down the mountain in a rainstorm as I suspect it would be pretty slick, like wet blacktop roads during a good storm.

Michael kept filling in the silence with his ongoing chatter while Carol and I concentrated on the job at hand. My eyes darting from this step to the next step. My poles choosing the best places to give me the best support possible, especially in tricky areas. And sometimes, I just had to take the poles in one hand and use my free hand to grab on to something – occasionally Michael's hand – to get up to the next step on the trail. Same for Carol. I knew how much energy it was taking to get my sorry butt up this mountain, but Carol was carrying an extra 100 pounds. I tried imagining me with a 100-pound Army pack on my back and how the degree of difficulty just increased by about a zillion percent. God love her, she never complained and still smiled often, despite breathing hard in the heat and with the work.

The walk was painfully slow, especially as the altitude increased with each step. Less air to breath. More pitch to lean into. We stopped about every 20 minutes, just long enough to catch our breath and wipe the sweat from our sunglasses. Michael's patience and encouragement keeping us going. After about an hour Carol sat down to rest but then took off one of her new hiking boots she'd bought specifically for the camp, tapping it as if to get something out of it.

"Something's in my shoe," she muttered as she pounded the boot onto the rock, awaiting some small pebble or other to come out, yet none did. She tipped it up to take a peek inside, but found nothing.

"Crap," she said. "I just got these since my other old beat-up ones looked like they wouldn't go another step and now these act up after I spent a pretty penny on them?" She rubbed the place on the back of her heel where it had been bothering her, pulled her socks tight in case that had anything to do with the problem, and was about to put the boot back on when Michael asked her to show him what brand of boot she'd bought.

"Great company. I highly recommend them. But how long did you take to break them in before you came?" he asked.

Carol looked worried then. "I didn't think I'd have to break them in. They have all that nice cushioning around the back and everything, and they felt so comfortable in the store." I could sense her becoming more concerned.

"Well," said Michael, "no second-guessing now. Not much we can do until we get back home. Just do your best to keep

 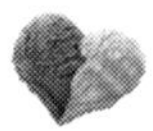

your sock pulled up taut so it doesn't have room to slip and slide in there. Keep your eyes on it and we'll play it by ear, OK? He smiled at her slightly frowning face and said, "Come on. We're half-way up." He gave her a hand up and we commenced again.

Not long after, Todd suddenly appeared out of nowhere. He and the guys had already hit the top and he'd come back down to see if Michael would like to check in with Jim and Chris for a while, offering himself to come "babysit" us. It was sweet of Todd to think of it and Michael took advantage of it in a heartbeat, for while he was dedicated to making sure all of us (namely us slow gals) were safe and having a good time, he was also cognizant of a great workout for himself when he saw one. He'd likely run the remaining half to the top full out, banging out about an extra 500 calories while also getting some serious glute and thigh work done with the pounding his legs would receive! He made sure we were OK with the plan, then headed out at a brisk jog, as predicted.

We spent the next hour or so with Todd in the lead and Carol and I slowly bringing up the rear. She, I knew, was worried about her heel and I was seriously conscious about where I stepped each time, remembering to keep my breathing steady and deep to get as much oxygen to my muscles and my brain that I could.

The pitch of the mountain seemed to become sharper by then and I spent little time looking down. (Did I mention that I'm not so keen on heights either?) With Todd's help I avoided some nasty spots and just kept my eyes peeled to where each step and each pole was going to end and start again. I'm not sure, but I'm guessing that if I hadn't had these people pushing me (once again) to my max, I'd have turned around long before then and simply said, "Nope. That's it for me." Which is what I had done in France on a family trip when my daughter was about 12 and we'd visited Paris and I would only go to the second highest level, not the very highest level, of the Eiffel Tower. I'd let fear hold me back then, much to the disappointment of my family, and looking back now, to myself as well.

I would NOT give up on this one.

Finally, unbelievably, thank-the-Lord-at-last, we hit the top and prayed whatever each of us prayed for getting us there. We were sure to thank Todd as well. He really had made us do a double-take on his earlier childish behavior. And he actually seemed to feel good about doing so himself. He'd let his ego take a hike by itself for a few minutes and finally relaxed into being just a kid. He just hadn't really found his way yet, despite his tough demeanor.

The view was breathtaking and at last I understood why no form of photo or video could capture it, although many had tried. There was just too much of it. So much pink granite that had been here in this upside-down Jello mold for centuries, and which would likely spend centuries more doing so ... the thought was absolutely mind-boggling.

It definitely felt enchanted, spiritual, or magical in some way. I could imagine some of the original explorers suddenly coming upon this strange place out in the middle of nowhere wondering just how to describe what they had found and why it was out here. On the other side of possibilities, one had to wonder if it had any alien links of some kind. OK, maybe no one mentioned it, but it would have been an interesting conversation.

 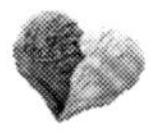

We perched at the edge of a shallow puddle with rather nasty looking rainfall water in it, but one that Carol was eyeing immediately for a way to soak her aching feet. We all were grateful to take a load off, and Carol especially. Unfortunately, however, when she removed her sock, the stinging pain was instant and she hissed through her teeth as the new blister showed it's red-faced ugliness to all who saw it.

Most of us did a quick peek and then glanced around at each other; the look in all our eyes saying, "Well, this isn't good." No one knew what to say for several seconds, then Carol broke the silence, "Well, let's see if that's the only one," and pulling off her other boot and sock she found the early stages of a young blister growing there as well. This one just hadn't started screaming yet. She sighed heavily and muttered, "And I thought I was doing myself a favor buying decent boots for all this hiking."

"Ouch." I said. Searching my mind for options. The long ago nurse side of me wanted to jump in and help in some way, but I had no supplies or ideas to pull from. It was going to be a long walk down. With a lot of pain ... and no Band-aids even.

Carol dug through her back pack and grabbed a couple of protein bars that we'd each brought for the trip. Apparently her appetite had won over the pain as she ripped open a bar and attacked it with zeal! That's one of the things I'd learned to like about Carol the last few days ... she doesn't seem to sweat the small stuff.

We'd taken nearly a couple of hours to get up there and it would likely take longer than that to get back down. Especially with Carol's new owies. But right now, with her boots off and feet soaking in the cool but rather nasty looking water, she didn't seem to have a worry in the world. She took in a huge breath, spread her arms to the sky as if thanking God for this most beautiful of places, and said, "This is just incredible."

The best the nurse in me could do was to have her use the bottled water we had to clean the blisters, then let them bake in the sun to dry for a bit, until we were ready to head down.

"There are Band-aids in the van in the first aid kit," Michael offered. "And when we get to the ranch I've got these amazing blister treatments pads that will get you back in the game with almost no pain, so I'll get you all set with them and you'll be good as new tomorrow." He sighed heavily, "Unfortunately, you'll have to get down the mountain first."

With Carol's attitude remaining upbeat, everyone seemed to relax as well, grabbing various goodies from their packs to fill their empty tummies. And the day was only halfway over.

Finally, after everyone had lunch, had taken a hundred pictures of the amazing place called Enchanted Rock, and had even grabbed a quickie power nap or two, it was time to face the music. We had to go back down.

Carol had gotten her socks and boots on again, although not easily. We all held our collective breath as she got up and started limping gingerly in the direction we had come up from, and despite the fact that we knew the damned little buggers must have stung like crap, she headed down the mountain without complaint.

I must admit that going down had me more worried than going up, and that worry proved to be valid. First of all, the pitch of the mountain seemed much steeper going down. I

 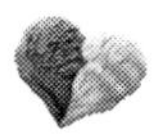

was definitely moving slower and more carefully. And of course, Carol was as well. We had also lost both Todd and Michael after lunch, as they wanted to check out a small cave a bit out of the way before we headed back. And since they were speed demons at mountain maneuvering, they should have been able to meet back up with us about half way down the rock. However, due to some miscalculations, and the mere size of the place, we got separated and Carol and I ended up with Chris and Jim hanging with us and glad for that. Except for one thing … they didn't know the path down either and the trail markers for the downhill directions didn't seem to be nearly as clear or as frequent.

Undaunted, we inched down the rock, bit by bit, all of us looking for the best trails to choose for the descent. Trails that didn't distinguish themselves often from the asphalt-like texture of the rock. Of course, it wasn't like we could get lost. Rather, it was like we were little ants on the face of a huge, cement wall for anyone to see. They wouldn't leave us out there all night clinging to a cold rock face in the dark! However, we were all exhausted and our brains were fried, so the odds of making some not-so-great decisions were probably pretty high. Between that and Carol's situation it paid for us to be extra careful.

Through a stressful and painstaking process we made it back and just before reaching the trail heads to the visitor center we ran into Michael and Todd, who had been looking for us as long as we'd been looking for them.

Michael apologized all over the place, especially to Carol and me who he knew he really needed to stay on top of. Unfortunately, they had missed out on reading some trail markers correctly themselves and had ended up as completely lost as we had been – and these were guys who'd actually been there before!

"How are your feet doing, Carol?" Michael inquired, worried. You could tell he was really embarrassed in both losing his teammates as well as not having tossed any Band-aids in his jeans for the hike.

Her face red (both from sunburn as well as being over-heated), Carol simply smiled and said, "I think I'm gonna need those Band-aids."

All in all, it was a day that kicked all of our butts but an adventure that wouldn't likely come our way again too often. While it worked both my body and Miss Mojo, almost too much, it was yet again another day where I put myself out there just a little farther than the day before, or the day before that.

What might I be able to do by the end of two weeks? Miss Mojo was curious too.

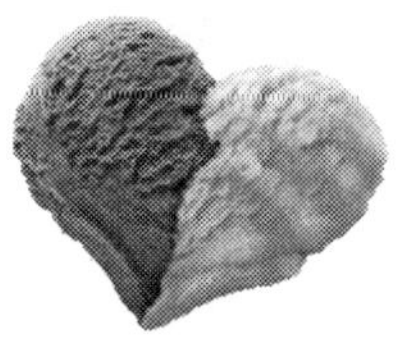

CHAPTER 25

My Road And The Obstacle Course

By about Thursday we had settled into our routines and most of our owies were healing nicely. Even the muscle cramps and general aches and pains of the workouts were abating.

Michael was true to his word about getting Carol locked and loaded again with his magic blister packs. He carefully trimmed the damaged skin from the blisters, then fitted some kind of gel onto some kind of contoured bandages that fit her feet just right, and sure enough, she was back in the saddle almost instantly.

On my end, I realized that I wasn't munching on Advil quite so often, so that was a definite improvement as well. Of course, I had also learned that the best plan for me at the end of each day was to eat dinner and walk my one-mile gravel road both ways to get to hear some friendly, encouraging voices from home. Then head to the small outdoor pool to cool down and watch the ever-present falling stars. Then wrap it all up by hanging out in the Jacuzzi with its hot, magic healing jets for as long as I could stand it. Then off to the bunkhouse to try to type up a few notes about the day. Then pray I could sleep, for 6:15 a.m. always seemed to come way too soon.

The others spent their evenings in different ways. Jim always hurried off to the bunkhouse to binge-watch *Game of Thrones* on his computer, so we didn't see much of him after dinner. Todd would watch TV if he hung around, although most nights he headed into town for whatever food or drink he could consume. I think he got friendly with one of the female camp employees as well, and they were looking for some privacy, definitely off-ranch. Carol spent her free time in the lounge on her computer. And if Chris didn't join me walking my road, he was likely hitting the hay early or else icing some body part in his room. Lil Deb mainly hung out in her room working on the communications she was having with that potential employer. In fact, she ended up leaving not long after our group finally got settled in, as the job looked like a pretty good opportunity and she'd done what she had hoped to accomplish at the ranch.

Most everyone thought I walked my gravel road (frequently with someone, but not always) just to make my phone call to my daughter every night, but honestly, it was also my dirty little secret. While these walks were only at an easy-going pace I set for myself, I knew that two miles per day was an extra 14 miles per week of calories burned. I just felt that I had to push myself in whatever way I could, without hurting my body unnecessarily. Extra walking was just walking, after all, but the calories burned kept adding up.

But, I had to admit to myself, it was more than just the calories. For some reason I just wanted to own this road. I

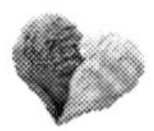

don't know if this need started that first night with the neck-and-neck race with Jim, or if it was just an old competitiveness in me left over from my athletic days, or maybe a way of feeling stronger instead of older … or something else completely. I didn't know. I just knew, for those nights, it was MY little corner of the world.

I even left the gym mid-afternoon one day when it was about as hot as it could get, and chose walking on my road over participating in the Zumba demonstration. I'd done Zumba at home at the gym and loved it, actually. But for some reason I just couldn't connect with the gal who'd come by special just to teach us and so I headed out. As always, it was waiting there for me. It felt like my go-to place. My safe place. The place I thought I would find some answers. So every night, alone or with someone, I trekked up that road at a relaxing pace. Not racing. Knowing by the end of my time there I should have been able to clock in 28 extra miles over anybody else; having accomplished more than a marathon even. And that was no number to laugh at.

It turned out to be so much more than that in the end.

***

One of my other favorite things that helped me in ways I hadn't predicted was the obstacle course. One morning while we were doing our pre-breakfast hike around the ranch, we walked through a part of the property that contained this obstacle course, something I hadn't heard was part of our activities and apparently was run on Saturdays by Michael's brother Gilbert, who was there on Michael's day off. It was clear that Lil Deb and Todd loved it, as they jumped in right away to show us the ropes. There were several obstacles to test various abilities, strength, and skills. Deb began by walking the telephone pole – mock "balance beam" – lying in the dirt. That looked easy as pie yet still required reasonable balance to navigate, even for only a handful of steps.

While she did that, Todd walked to the end of a gigantic chain that weighed a ton, picked up the loose end of it, then turned around so that it was swung across his back. From there, he took off running as fast as he could, hauling the massive chain behind him. When he'd finished, he turned again and faced the chain, pulling its length through his legs, hand over hand, until it all was piled at his feet again. I was correct in assuming the task was much more difficult than he made it look.

Next they demonstrated the giant tire – the size that fits on a tractor or something even larger. The object there was to flip the tire over and over again for a certain distance. (I knew my spinal surgeon would kill me for that one so I eliminated it from the start!) Todd had begun to flip the tire and once he got his rhythm, was moving the heavy thing quite effectively, despite the beads of sweat rolling down his face and into his eyes so he could barely see.

Next, there were the free-floating stairs. I'm sure there's a name for them, but basically it was a staircase about three or four feet off the ground that you went up one side and down the other; the tricky part was that the stairs appeared suspended in air somehow. It was probably more of an optical illusion than anything but it was definitely attention-getting and required some balance. Deb obviously liked this one and had become quite good at it during her stint here.

 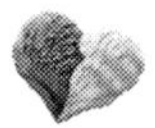

Then, on to the classic tire test, with two rows of standard-size tires running parallel to each other and the participant steps left into one tire then right into the next. (You see that one in almost every football movie ever made.) Todd showed us all how nimble he was, running up and back down the thing as graceful as any ballerina. (Although he would have been horrified to hear me say that!) And then there was the sled skill, consisting of a flat wooden palate stacked with heavy wood that you dragged behind you attached to a rope around the waist. Todd slipped into that rope too and leaned his whole body into the pull, dragging it very slowly but a hell of a lot farther than I knew I'd be doing anytime soon!

I saw that there were a few other smaller ones that weren't a big deal, but there was one that had both Carol and me just a tad nervous. It was a two-parter: on the one side was a piece of plywood, sloped at 45 degrees, leaning up against a sturdy wall of four by fours. A heavy cotton climbing rope was attached to the top. On the adjacent side was a ladder like you'd find in a hay barn, with wide, sturdy planks. The whole piece stood about eight or nine feet high.

The object was to grab the rope and climb that piece of slippery plywood, pulling yourself up the line until you reached the top, where there were very few things to hold on to. Then, IF you made it that high, you had to climb up and over the top, then climb down the ladder on the other side to the ground. For those who knew how to do it, they made it *look* easy, although it was clearly not. Deb and Todd both loved the thing, you could tell. They each must have climbed it at least twice, laughing and joking with each other as they did so. Looking like a couple of monkeys on the monkey bars.

Chris and Jim took their turns when the first two seemed to get their fill. Chris had certainly been on something like it in boot camp or other military training school, and flew up it nimbly, despite the added weight around his middle. Jim gave it a go as well and had no complaint. He got it on the first try.

I wasn't sure if Carol was intimidated by it and didn't think she could do it, or was worried about the physical work involved in getting herself over the contraption … but she was definitely worried. Her usual cheery voice had grown silent.

I, on the other hand, always loved doing something like this. It took me back to all the playgrounds I'd been on in my lifetime and our gymnastics classes in high school, all which I had absolutely loved back in the day. But these days my fear factor involving medical issues were screaming at me. Could I possibly wreck my back (further) doing this? Was it worth it? Or was I just counting up my excuses?

I lucked out for the moment as it was time for breakfast, but Saturday would arrive soon and I'd have to decide what I was comfortable doing.

***

It was the end of another very long day and I was desperately trying to keep my eyes open long enough to type a few notes about the day's events – especially my worries about the obstacle course. Those original worry buds had grown into dancing little nightmare glimpses of me sliding backwards down the slippery plywood ramp, frantically scrambling to

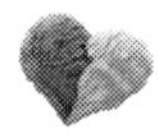

keep my balance but watching myself, as if in slow motion, back pedaling to save my life. Then slipping one last time and falling in a huge, motionless heap on the ground. Followed by a horrific image of everyone trying to help me but realizing they needed to call in some Flight For Life rescue team to haul me off to some trauma center instead; everyone wondering if I'd ever walk again. I think I might have even been able to imagine the view of the world outside of the helicopter from my front row, sky vantage seat stretcher but thank God Carol broke that train of thought.

"Hey, MJ, can I ask you something," she inquired softly from her bed. She too had been off her feed all day and her usual effervescence had disappeared since the morning's demonstration.

"Sure," I answered, "what's up?" Of course I suspected her brain was on a similar path to mine but I couldn't have anticipated what she'd been brewing on all day.

She squirmed a bit before asking, "Do you think Chris would help me?"

"Help you with what?" I queried. I wasn't in a place I could look her in the face to get a read on what was going on. But there was something in her voice that told me this could be a make or break moment for her too.

She started out slowly but then as her thoughts started making more and more sense to her, she gradually increased her wordy communication until it was nearly a flood. "With that thing on the obstacle course. You know which one I'm talking about." Of course I did.

"Well, I was thinking that – you know – he's been in the military and all. He knows this stuff. And you saw how he sailed right over that damned slip-slidey board, almost as if it were a skating rink and he was on skates, zooming around like he'd done it all his life. Making it look so ... ah ... well ... blooming easy!" I could tell she wished she could use a more powerful word, but swearing did not come with her Evangelical upbringing.

"Yeah, he sure did," I concurred. Envious as hell of him as well. I wanted to be that athletic and strong. And sure. He was so confident in himself. I think the missing confidence factor played as big a part as anything for us. It wasn't like we could just go out and buy some confidence, especially not way out here in the boonies.

"What do you have in mind, exactly?" I was definitely interested by then. She had obviously been thinking about this all day.

"Well," she sighed, forging on. "I'd just like to see if he wouldn't take me up there after we're done for the day and teach me one-on-one so that by the time Saturday is here I don't look like an idiot in front of everybody."

Smart.

"Sure, Carol. I bet he'd be glad to help you. Maybe me too. I'm a little shaky about it myself. How about if we ask him in the morning?"

I could feel her smile returning even though I couldn't see her face.

***

We kept the plan just between us three, heading up the hillside to the obstacle course after a long day of activities once again.

 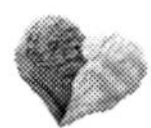

It almost felt like we were covert operatives or something, sneaking off from the others when they weren't watching.

Of course Chris was wide open to the idea. Carol rightly figured that he'd likely done a lot of teaching in his years with the military and his amiable nature was a perfect calm for anyone with a few nerves leaving them shaking and quaking.

"OK, guys," he lead off, "the biggest thing to remember is that it's about momentum, momentum, momentum. There is no stopping. Only going forward. Got that?" He looked back and forth at us, his eyes telling us that we weren't going to get out of this now, come hell or high water. I felt myself gulp and looked to Carol, whose face had suddenly seemed to turn robotic, like some Marvel Comic super-hero or something. She'd come wearing her workout gloves from the gym and suddenly stopped and stripped them off and threw them on the ground, all the while staring at "It." The elephant in the room. The thing we feared so much that we didn't even have a name for it.

She walked over to It and grabbed the heavy, cotton rope in both hands and perched her right foot on the dreaded plywood as Chris started his step-by-step, melodic directions with a good dose of cheerleading thrown in. "OK, now, deep breath, Carol. (Breath.) You know what you've got to do. (Breath.) You're going to go all the way to the top and keep going. (Breath.)" And suddenly she dug in with all her might and launched herself up that ramp – focused, determined, unstoppable.

"That's it, dig in, dig in," I found myself cheering her as well, as I watched her winning the battle. Chris was still shouting at her, "Go, go, go," as she reached for the top, easily balancing on the highest bar before she had to go down the other side with the ladder. It had only taken about three big steps and three small ones to make it up there, but they seemed to be some of the biggest ones of her life.

"Stop for a pose at the top," I reminded her, as I'd been in charge of recording the event. She turned to face me, did her best Popeye pose, showing off both her muscles and her pride, then started climbing down the ladder back to Terra Firma.

"Too strong!" shouted Chris. "How strong are you, Carol? Too strong!" It had a sound reminiscent of the Marine's "Hoo Rah!"

"And you made it look easy breezy to boot!" I could sense his pride in making it happen.

She was beaming when she hit the ground. And I was so happy for her. For not only was that a big emotional boost accomplishing something so daunting, she did it carrying more weight than anyone else at camp. In essence, no one worked as hard as Carol did at succeeding at the task.

"I want to do that again!" She laughed. "I was so afraid of it and now I want to do it again!" She turned and stared at "It", hoping it hadn't all been a figment of her imagination, but I reassured her that I had it all on tape, and held up my iPhone for her to watch the events again. She was still huffing and puffing but I hadn't seen her happier than that moment all week.

"Next," shouted Chris. And I knew he meant me.

The good thing was that Carol had had success, and made it look like a piece of cake. But of course, I was also a few decades older than her and pretty much held together with titanium, nuts and bolts, and God knows what. I remember

 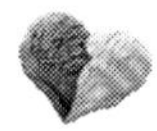

asking my spinal surgeon when he cleared me for most activities, after all my months of surgery and rehab, if I could return to horseback riding again. His answer was simple: "Sure, just don't fall off." His voice in my head seemed to be awfully loud that day.

Yet, here I was, with the best team of buds to help me reach just a little bit farther today than yesterday. People who seemed willing to help me find yet another crumb of my Mojo, playing out here in the desert with "It," all the while still searching for their own answers as well. I trusted these people and I'd only known them a handful of days. I felt safe with them. I knew I could do it.

We all moved closer to "It" once again and I reached for the cotton rope, my gloved hands sweating to beat the band underneath the neoprene. I took a huge gulp of air then blasted off, taking three strong, determined steps up the plank followed by three small ones that got me a toe-hold at the top, as my cheerleaders clapped and whooped and shouted words I didn't even hear. (I watched the video afterwards and realized they were saying things like, "Come on, come on, come on." (Chris) Or "You're amazing, you go girl." (Carol). But the only voice I heard was the little one in my head that said, "Use your Mojo. What are you waiting for?"

I felt like Dorothy in *The Wizard of Oz* realizing she was already in Kansas and could quit looking for home elsewhere.

As I climbed down the ladder they both engulfed me in a huge group hug, shrieking and hollering as if my success was their success as well. And of course, it was. Carol and I each climbed It a couple of more times to cement the deal in our minds, as well as in our muscle memory. And we indeed surprised everyone at Saturday's obstacle day when we sailed through the activities with more confidence than anyone anticipated.

And even now, two years after camp, Carol, Chris, and I still touch base occasionally. I've never heard from anyone else.

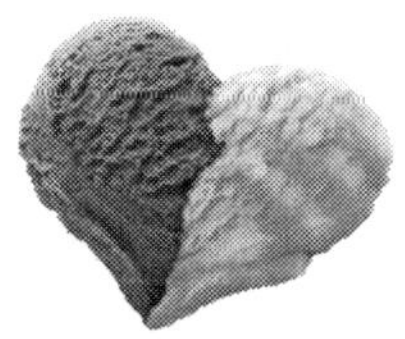

CHAPTER 26

The Wrap Up

The days took on a natural flow. The Wake Up workout. Breakfast and morning workouts or hikes. Lunch. Afternoon workouts. Power naps during our short breaks. Water aerobics. Dinner. My walk to the mailbox. Admiring shooting stars almost every night by the little pool. Soaking in the hot tub to get the tired muscles to let go of the stress of the day. Falling into bed so exhausted sometimes I still couldn't sleep. And barely sneaking in a few notes of the day to my computer's memory banks so I didn't forget anything.

While we were getting stronger day by day, some of our chronic aches and pains never seemed to cut us a break. Chris, for example, wore his knee brace all the time, and I suspected his knee was still killing him more than he let on. It appeared that it had been giving him trouble for years, so it wasn't going to go away anytime soon. But it definitely limited his abilities to do things, which likely bothered him as much as, if not more than, the pain.

Then a really crazy thing happened to Chris while we were doing Yoga one afternoon. We'd been doing some kind of arm work before Yoga and apparently he had strained something in his elbow, quite unknowingly. Then, when he lay flat on the floor to do Yoga, some joint fluid must have found a new, little space between his overstretched muscles and began pooling in the space at the end of his elbow. He suddenly looked like his elbow was giving birth to a tennis ball! I mean, picture some movie about aliens where some part of some creature from outer space suddenly sprouts a new creature by leaking it out of their elbow joint. It was just about that creepy and scared us all to death.

The look on Chris' face was one I don't think I'll ever forget. While he knew all those alien movies were make believe, at that moment in time, the possibility of an alien birth taking place from his elbow suddenly seemed like a real possibility! "What the hell is it? My God, what the hell is it?" he was yelling as we all ran up to see the phenomenon. And sure enough, it looked like an alien-elbow birth to all of us. And the "infant" had instantly grown from the size of a golf ball to a tennis ball in a matter of moments.

Michael was off that day and the poor yoga teacher was out of her league. I asked her about the nearest medical facilities, which she said was a bit of a drive away. With Chris freaking out I didn't think he'd handle it any better with a 30-minute car ride to an ER, so I took a chance and called my daughter at work in Missouri for her orthopedic surgeon insights and did a quick consult. Fortunately she happened to pick up the phone on the first ring and I was so grateful. Then she told me to take a photo of it and text it to her. Within minutes she allayed all our fears. She assured us that he'd be fine with ice and rest, and not to do any more workouts for the day. I took pictures of that one! Can you say "ugly"?

On a more chronic, less exciting topic, my back (surprise, surprise) was a constant source of my usual chronic bunch of knots I dealt with at home on a regular basis but even more so pushing them here. I was glad I'd brought both my biggest bottle of Advil and Tylenol, and was popping them as much as allowed on the label.

I think Todd twisted his ankle about Thursday and he tried to milk himself some sympathy from it but since most of us were nursing war wounds of our own, he didn't get much.

Whenever Chris walked the gravel road with me to call his girlfriend we sort of touched base about how we were feeling about the upcoming end of our visit – namely, our follow-up race of The Mile. As the day grew closer he groaned whenever we spoke of it, as if reliving the pain he'd experienced the first time and essentially told me he had nothing to prove this time. He was in enough pain that he didn't think it was worth adding to it. He was just going to walk and leave it at that.

I figured he was right about that. However, I wasn't sure exactly where I was standing on the topic yet. Sure, my back hurt. And my titanium knees were chronically achy – considering what I'd asked of these body parts at camp, I was more than pleased with them, actually. While I still was going to follow doctors orders and not jog or run any length of The Mile, Miss Mojo was already suggesting that I wanted to own that road. I'd earned it all week, walking the extra two miles of it each and every night. Even alone sometimes. It was as though I'd claimed my territory – and myself – back through that dry, dusty road. I wondered how it would play out.

***

There was one very disappointing note for me that took place at the end of week one. It was time for the one-week weigh-in and we were all excited and scared to death at the same time. We'd worked our bodies in ways we'd never dreamed possible and had the aches and pains and blisters and strains to prove it.

We'd also stayed pretty much on track, food-wise. At least up to the weigh-in. Todd had his own plans for after the weigh-in that we'd hear about later.

I do have to confess to stealing three or four chocolate chip cookies from the kitchen after hours during the week. Plus I did have a *s'more* at the campfire one night, among the dudes and dudettes, who didn't care a lick what I put in my mouth. But for the most part, especially combined with four hours working out per day, I was optimistic of a decent number. Of course I also kept forgetting that no one but me had already been in a regular workout regimen prior to coming, nor was anyone but me only 15 or so pounds away from goal – important keys to factor in to just how much weight loss was possible.

We all hung out in the lounge and one by one took our turn privately with Michael, in his office … where the dreaded scale lived. Jim went first and came out with a small smile, reporting four pounds dropped. We all whooped up a storm for him and he was clearly pleased, then plopped himself back down in a chair while the others took their turns before we headed out for the morning hike.

Next, Carol, hesitant but optimistic. She returned quickly with a huge smile: 7-1/2 pounds. Chris was next with another 7 pounds, followed by Todd's 4. Smiles, applause, and congratulations for all.

At last it was my turn and I stepped on the scale, eyes closed, holding my breath, cautiously optimistic. When at last I opened my eyes, I let out in a huge gasp! ONE POUND! The damned scale said I'd only lost one pound!

My heart leapt to my throat and I almost couldn't breathe. That couldn't be right! For God's sake I could have lost that at home just not eating for a day! And here I'd burned more calories in a week than in most months and for what? I had to really suck it up not to cry and, although Michael knew I was disappointed, I'm sure he had no idea just *how* disappointed I really was. All I could think of was how the price of one pound cost me $1,000.

"Don't worry, MJ," Michael put his arm around my shoulders, feeling the tension in them flooding in by the minute. "You don't have a ton of weight to lose like those folks. Your body is thinking that it needs to hold on to its weight right now as it gets down to what will be a new normal for you. Just stay the course. You're doing great."

I nodded my head, gave him a pretty fake smile and, barely keeping my tears under control, ventured back out to my awaiting teammates eager to hear how I did. Needless to say, I wasn't very talkative and headed out the door, hoping to stave off the tears.

I had never worked my body so hard in my whole life. How on Earth could I not do better than 1 pound? I immediately wanted to stuff my face with whatever crap I could find. Fortunately nothing was available to binge on and we were all heading out for a long hike day, so I just had to stuff my emotions for the time being, and get back to work. I avoided everyone most of the day and sat around feeling sorry for myself … as if that were going to fix anything.

Finally, when it was time to walk my road, I got back in the groove. Chris joined me and he spent the time giving me a pep talk about how it should all be about the long game. How one week in the grand scheme of things meant very little. How it was all about staying the course, sticking it out, and making it a healthy lifestyle, not just a diet. And he was right.

But I do still find it remarkable how one silly number can have so much power over us. If we let it. Thanks, guys, for teaching me that.

Todd had his own thoughts on the subject, however. His theory was that he had one "cheat day" every week that he could eat anything he wanted and would still lose weight. In fact, I think his mission was to get into the Guinness Book of Records under the heading of the most food consumed in an average day.

To demonstrate, he proudly boasted his cheating day's intake starting with a huge breakfast with pancakes and syrup, bacon, biscuits and gravy, and scrambled eggs. Lunch was a huge burger and fries from the food made for the dudes, with a couple of beers he'd brought from the bunkhouse. For dinner, he ended up eating three separate meals as he'd gone into town with Jim to get some real food. Then, upon returning to the ranch, and realizing that it was BBQ night in the mess hall, he filled himself up there. Yet, he didn't end there. As it turned out, it was the night Michael cooked something special for us; a fabulous salmon dinner, huge kale salad, and green beans. Todd decided that looked good as well and made himself a big plate. To top everything off, he indulged in two pieces of cherry pie for dessert, chased down with a six-pack of beer. And finally, having met a couple of cool guys from

London in the hot tub with a big bottle of tequila, he'd downed his share of that too, as they sat up until 3 a.m. learning about each other's culture. We all watched in awe, wondering just what his weight loss could possibly be after another week, at the rate he was eating. My stomach hurt just thinking about all the food he inhaled. And I was still reeling from the one pound weight loss. It was a bit hard to take.

***

At last, it was time for the final testing. The Mile, Part 2. I had been picturing this all week. Wondering what would happen this time. Wondering if I'd improved at all. Wondering, too, what everyone else was thinking as well. It almost seemed anti-climactic after everything else that had happened in two weeks, and yet it was a true black and white measurement of the new strength we all seemed to be developing. We lined up one last time, Carol knowing she'd still take up the rear but only caring to learn just how much she had improved. Todd was sitting this one out, since he'd been eating so much that day it probably wouldn't be wise to let him run it if he'd wanted to. That left just Jim, Chris, and me. And Chris's bad knee that had caught him by the tail last time.

We were eager to go and Michael's, "Ready, set, go," set us off once again. Jim and I quickly fell into our fast-paced walk but there was a new feeling of competitiveness you could cut with a knife, especially when we both watched Chris suddenly start jogging at a very fast clip, pulling away from us easily.

All of a sudden everything changed. Our competitive personalities had had two weeks to prepare for this little test that meant so much, and despite talking to the contrary every day beforehand – talking about taking it easy on his knee, nothing to prove to anyone – Chris apparently had to prove something after all.

I couldn't believe it. Miss Mojo was definitely returning, that much I knew. Because what I really wanted to do was jog with him neck and neck and really see who was going to kick whose butt! Jim was surprised too, but he just kept up our steady pace, content to improve his time without being stupid about it.

I decided that what my knee surgeon didn't know couldn't hurt him and I started a slow jog of my own – something that felt pretty much a reach, since I hadn't done that in nearly three years. And the last time was on the knees I was born with. I noticed that as Chris had progressed down the road he'd slowed to a quick walk, pacing himself. I decided that would be a good time to push myself and see if I couldn't catch him while he caught his breath. Yet as soon as I started jogging, he resumed jogging as well, and I cursed him under my breath. Son of a bitch! What happened to all those nights walking the road talking about not pushing ourselves like crazy people? What happened to his aching knee? Had he planned this all along or was this a last minute decision?

Well, none of it mattered. What mattered was what I did about it.

We were about half-way down the road by then and the sweat was rolling off us all … mine, at least, running in my eyes. At times I could barely see. I had to blink a few times to even get my contacts clear enough to see Chris still ahead of me, walking again, as he saw me return to my walking as well.

Jim was way behind me by then and I'd all but forgotten about him.

There was only my friend Chris. Chris who had helped me learn how to do the obstacle course. Chris who had walked with me so many nights on that very gravel road we had grown to know so well. Chris who I'd almost delivered an alien baby for during his camp crisis only days before. I could not let him win. I pushed on.

With only a few moments to go, I talked to Miss Mojo and said, "If ever there was a time to raise your strong you that's buried in there somewhere, this would be it." And I pushed myself to jog as fast as I could, huffing and puffing into a rhythm I hoped would bring me as much air as possible in that humid land. And I started gaining on him.

He looked back again, only this time his expression changed when he saw the new me heading straight for him. And I could see that this time he was worried. He tried to jog faster but I knew the knee had to be screaming at him by then. And I put my head down and pulled from everything I had.

By the last 20 yards I was puffing up his back and for a moment he turned and with the utmost respect, smiled. More like grinned, actually. As if almost apologizing for changing the plan at the last minute.

"See you at the finish line," I replied. And with the last bit of Mojo I could muster, I beat him by about 10 seconds!

The audience, consisting of Michael, Todd, the cook and the dishwasher kid, woo-hooed, and congratulated both of us as we reached for water they offered. Then we all turned back to watch Jim come in next, followed by Carol, who was making her steady way, obviously faster than the first time we were all here. It was a huge success. Everyone improved their times. I don't recall any specific times but it was the improvement that counted and which I remembered long after the race was over. And my knees were barely complaining. Thank you, knees. I promise not to do that again to you, at least not for a while.

I could hardly stand still once the race was over, I was so full of adrenaline. The road was mine! It was mine! I wanted to call it Mary Jo's Road. Or even better, for those who followed, Mojo Road. Because despite the fact that I shaved nearly two minutes off my time, the gift I came away with was discovering that little Miss Mojo, had never really been lost. She'd just been laying low for awhile, waiting for me to figure my life out. But this trip, this time, this road had let her become a huge part of my life again. "Welcome back, Darlin'."

***

The next day, as I said goodbye to everyone at the ranch I also said a little prayer to God thanking Him for pushing me out of my comfort zone to attend the ranch to begin with. It had seemed like a lot of money when I had a perfectly good gym I attended regularly at home. However, I would have never tested my physical limits like that anywhere else! Leave it to God to remember that I learn best through adventures I never see coming. From the dude ranch to Cozumel to Rancho Cortez, all had changed me in ways I could never have believed possible.

I was also really pleased that I had been able to keep up with the physical experiences at the ranch most of the time, during my time there, despite my body being held together by a wing and a prayer.

I was even OK with the environment – it was indeed rustic but as I was only in my room to sleep and change clothes, it was fine. I appreciated that there were various levels to choose from.

As to our weight losses … we all lost after two weeks. Carol and Chris lost 10# each. Jim and Todd, 8. And I, the thinnest of the bunch, lost 4.5 It wasn't as much as I'd hoped for but it came with lots of perks. I had lost some weight but gained so much.

***

Carol and Chris drove me to the airport where we hugged all around, knowing what a special time it had meant to all of us. "Good luck, you guys," I said, as I hugged them both. "Stay in touch and kick some more butt these next two weeks."

"Take care, MJ." Carol smiled one of her usual happy-as-a-lark smiles. She really was like a cherub sometimes. "Keep doing it, girl."

Chris just beamed at me, probably remembering my help with the alien elbow birth the most. "You're amazing. So glad I got to meet you."

I grabbed my suitcase and headed back home.

Yet one more unpredictable thing happened while I was still in the airport waiting for my flight that gave me the biggest smile of the whole damned trip ... I headed to grab some grub from one of the airport bars and, looking over the mostly fried foods and otherwise non-healthy items that dominated the menu, I decided that I really should at least attempt something healthy after all we'd learned – and after leaving $2,000 behind for my education.

After some study, I chose the salmon burger and a salad, minus the bun. Which was delicious, by the way. I think just the thought of it being real food for starters got my juices flowing and I'm sure I inhaled it all with an expression of satisfaction that can be attained through only one of a few things. I closed my eyes, savoring each bite. Even enjoying the odd lot drip that slipped down my chin, necessitating numerous napkins to keep up to it.

Having been busy with the relationship I was having with my dinner, I hadn't noticed a gentleman who had sat down near me at the bar. He'd apparently been watching me carry on like a homeless person with his first meal in weeks and asked, "So whatever it is you're eating, it must be amazing by the look on your face."

I opened my eyes, a bit embarrassed, and still wiping slobber down my face. I hadn't been approached by any unknown bar guy in as long as I could remember, and wasn't exactly sure what to say, especially until I could swallow that mouthful of food. And so, for that moment, I just shook my head, hoping that he'd figure out that he'd have to carry on the conversation for a moment until I could breathe.

"What is it, anyway?" he inquired, as my mouth finally emptied.

"Salmon burger," I replied. Smiling. After all, it felt kind of special being hit on, just leaving boot camp where I'd been soaked in nothing but sweat for two weeks solid.

The man made a face that said he was confused. "If it's a salmon burger, where's the bun?" By this time the piece of meat on my plate was so eaten that it really didn't resemble much of anything, so I understood his confusion.

Finally getting a decent speaking voice back I replied, "I told the bartender to hold the bun," I said. "Just shaved a few calories that way." I felt so proud that I hadn't ordered the greasy fish and chips, which had originally been my first choice.

His face looked really confused. And I could sense him give me another look-over, of as much of my body as he could see from our positions in our bar stools.

"Why on Earth should you worry about calories?" He genuinely didn't understand. "You look just perfect to me."

All I can say is, Thank you, Rancho Cortez. $2,000 well spent!

> PS. Since I left the ranch, I have dropped nearly fifteen pounds. Although they didn't all just leave right away.

BOOT CAMP DETAILS FOR THE BEST TIME POSSIBLE

Should you decide to venture out to your own fitness boot camp in the great outdoors, here's just a few tips:

- Give yourself as much time as possible to prepare. Doing a couple of thirty-minute rounds of slow and steady treadmill work at the gym each week is not enough to prepare for the amount of work a body will be doing with several workouts per day.

- Take your favorite forms of Icy Hot or Ben Gay and lots of Advil and Tylenol for all the aches and pains you will definitely experience. Bring LOTS!
- Do not take new hiking boots. Your favorite, beat-up old ones might be better. Or at least, if you've got to buy new ones get them far enough ahead of time to break them in well. Also, take plenty of Band-aids and a blister healing product, just in case.
- Take two really good pairs of tennis shoes. One pair can be drying out while you're wearing the other.
- Bring lots of sunscreen and bug spray.
- A flashlight with new batteries is helpful. It can get dark under those big, night skies.
- If phone availability is super important to you, get one of those enhanced Internet phones – especially if you don't want to walk the driveway every night to use the phone.
- Don't go in August unless you need a kick in the butt like I did. Sure, it's a dry heat. But 95 degrees on a bust-your-butt hike, is still 95 degrees!
- If you're really, really out of shape (haven't exercised at least a part of every day for some time) I highly suggest you start a walking program first. When you're feeling strong walking for an hour per day then go hang out at a gym for a month or two, in addition to the walking. Try out an elliptical,

treadmill, bike – whatever, just start to get your heart used to the idea of kicking up the pace a little.

- If you have constipation issues take plenty of laxative or fiber or whatever keeps thing moving, so to speak, as introducing all this healthy food to your body can be tough on your gut.

- Of course a video camera of some type is priceless. The folks at home will never believe the things you accomplish at this camp and you'll need the video to prove it.

- A journal or computer to jot down thoughts about your experiences. I never would have remembered half of our crazy and fun experiences without one!

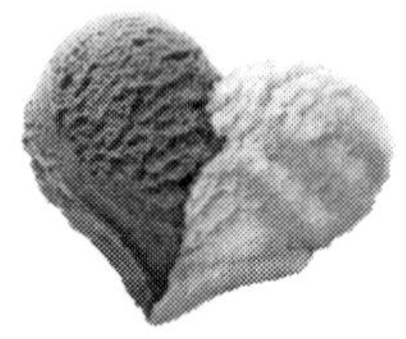

CHAPTER 27

No Cheatin', Just Eatin'

I returned to Colorado feeling refreshed and excited about my experiences at the ranch. But I still hadn't found my direction yet. I was getting tired of being a relationship coach. I'd led the Denver Dating, Mating, and Relating Meetup group for ten years. While the group had been an overwhelming success with a great reputation, and I had married several couples who had met through the group, it didn't excite me any more. In addition, new, younger dating coaches were taking Denver by storm with enough energy to run rings around me as well.

I was still doing some individual coaching – a few for dating help and I still continued to help a few who were mired in a relationship with some abusive narcissist or other, desperate for help. Yet, the hard part with helping most of them was that they were often so messed up from the manipulation they'd lived with for so long that, while they talked about wanting to leave their abusers, they always returned to them. In the end, all the negativity was just too hard to watch and brought way too much negative energy my way. I just couldn't handle so many pessimistic people. They had a way of zapping

 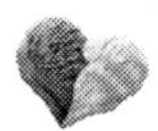

my energy, and these days, I just didn't have any extra to spare. I needed to take care of myself first.

I ached to find some new direction, yet nothing appealed to me. And Miss Mojo was quiet. Not because she was unhappy with me, but because she usually was the cheerleader once a new idea would leap into my head. Coming up with the creative idea was my responsibility. In all my other books or projects, it had always happened that way for me. Bang! Some idea would just pop up and would suddenly make sense and I would latch onto it for all it was worth.

When it came to writing a book, however, once I got the idea clearly in my head I would immerse myself and do nothing but write until the project was done, usually in a couple of months. I'd work from morning until the wee hours of the night, with energy just pouring out of me. And if there was a time crunch for some reason, even better. All my life I had always done best under pressure.

I'd kind of dabbled with the idea of writing a book about Rancho Cortez but I didn't really have enough to write an entire book just about that. Something still seemed missing, so I wasn't going to jump on that until I could envision it.

Months went by and 2014 turned into 2015 with me still going through the motions. I did stay active at the gym. At least I hadn't left that behind. It had become part of my daily routine. And, with my new outlook, I'd been able to keep my weight in the mid-160's without having to track absolutely everything. (I was content to be in maintenance mode, not losing mode.) Not great, but not bad. Or as I often still tried to convince myself, just "Not that bad."

I also had a group of friends at the gym so it was a piece of my social life as well. Bernie was still around and we'd always banter a bit, teasing and cheerleading whenever we crossed paths. I missed Mary Ann like crazy and actually spent ten days with her in Oregon when she had a hip replaced. And although we spoke by phone almost daily, it wasn't the same as having her just a five-minute drive away. She'd been my closest "go to gal," and now she was miles and miles away.

Then suddenly, a series of events took place that changed everything, starting with my rent going up – again. With the legalization of marijuana in Colorado, many more people were moving there, driving real estate values through the roof. My landlord again raised my rent on my two bedroom, two bath house to $1,450 per month. I couldn't afford to live there any more.

At the same time, my daughter was finally finishing fourteen years of training to become an orthopedic trauma surgeon and had taken a position fulfilling that role in Topeka, Kansas. In the ten years prior, I generally only saw her for a handful of days each year. The life of a surgical resident is such that they barely get time off to eat and sleep, much less have a real life. Now, as an attending doctor, on the top of the food chain, she would finally have a semi-normal life, not only getting time to spend with her family, but with me too!

I always knew that I'd end up living close to her at some point – I just didn't expect it to all happen as suddenly as it did. Nor did I imagine it would be in Kansas.

I drove out from Denver to attend her final graduation from her trauma fellowship and thought I'd just check out a few houses to see what the market was like, and in a matter of four days I'd put a contract on a house. And by mid-September I was settling into my new home in Topeka.

I spent more time with my daughter in those first two weeks than I had in the previous 14 years! I couldn't have been happier with the situation.

It took me a few weeks to get the boxes emptied and the house put together. And man did I keep my body working out throughout that process. Going up and down stairs to the attic and the basement several times per day, several days in a row, my knees were holding out fine. But I was shocked when, a few weeks later, I weighed myself in at 159#. I hadn't seen that number since the post-wedding days when I was working out like a crazy person and before my back went to hell in a hand basket. And I hadn't been tracking my food for ages, with all that had been going on. I'd kind of let 165 or so be my baseline weight, secretly convinced that I just wasn't able to get any lower than that anyway. Yet, still seeing that number in my doctor's office chart as falling into the Overweight category.

Yet, there it was – 159#. My heart went thump, thump and Miss Mojo smiled and I decided perhaps it was time to push the edge of the envelope again. Could I lose those last few pounds and make 150 or so my new baseline? Was there a chance that I could turn back time to my high school weight of 148, back in the days when I ran on the track team?

As I considered this idea I realized one important key: I wasn't at the 100-percent intention stage. There was no big class reunion or another wedding or any other event coming that would drive me to work out again as hard as I had in 2009. Nor did I want to work out that hard, ever again. But maybe I could develop a project out of it somehow. And maybe I'd not only help me, I'd find a way to help others as well.

Of course, my doctor was always reminding me that I could slow down the progression of my illness by exercising as often as possible. It was the least I could do for myself. I didn't even need a gym membership, honestly. I could simply go for a walk if that's what made the most sense. (Although for me, the hot tub at a gym was well worth the price of $22 per month alone.)

So, I got my tracking calendar back up on the wall, my journal set up for tracking calories-in and calories burned, and Shaun bought me a Misfit tracker for Mother's Day, with all the bells and whistles that the Body Bug didn't have in its day. And I could even get it wet. Then I went shopping for a gym and ended up joining the YWCA. I was back in business and ready to see just how low I could go.

One of the first things I found was a water volleyball league that played three days a week for two hours. Sounded awesome! I showed up one day and they welcomed me in. Little did I know that these mostly senior citizens were butt-kicking, take-no-prisoners volleyball players. You'd think they were trying out for the Olympics, that's how seriously they took the game, although they could laugh at themselves as well when goofy stuff happened throughout the game, as it always did.

I took up playing with them six hours a week and loved it. Both the game and the people. They even had lunch together after every game and invited me along. I started making some friends.

One thing that felt very different from Denver, however, was that people kept asking me if I was a model or a marathon runner. I think one even called me Twiggy. Me? A model?

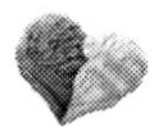

Twiggy? What *were* they talking about? I was still carrying around those damned extra pounds that still classified me as overweight and that just wouldn't go away. I sure didn't feel like Twiggy in my size 14's.

And then I remembered that Colorado touts the lowest obesity statistics in the whole country. On any given day people are running, biking, skating, skiing, playing tennis or basketball, dancing, working out at the gym; the list goes on. Colorado even claims to have the third highest (per capita) number of SCUBA divers in the US and they're nowhere near an ocean. These people live and breathe fitness! Every day of the year. No excuses.

When it came to food and nutrition, while my Colorado friends made kale a mainstay, my Kansas friends looked at it as if it were some kind of alien plant. In fact, I attended a funeral and stayed for the luncheon, which was loaded with the usual Kansas fare – fried chicken, tater tots, dinner rolls, mac and cheese, coleslaw, baked beans, a gorgeous kale salad with everything but the kitchen sink in it, and cake for dessert. While all the other foods disappeared in a heartbeat, the poor kale salad remained largely untouched. I devoured it as if it were the main course. It was absolutely the best salad I'd ever had in my life! I couldn't believe no one else was eating it. The good news? The nice church ladies said I could take the enormous salad home, if I wanted to. Jackpot! I ate almost nothing but that salad for three days.

My experience at that funeral made me realize that I wasn't in Colorado anymore, Toto. The Kansas culture around food was entirely different from what I was used to ... not even with my horrible nutrition. Food was a social essential.

Fitness was not. In this world, I did stick out as if I were Twiggy. While that felt good, it also suggested to people that I was one of those naturally skinny people who could eat whatever I wanted and never gain an ounce. The ones they hated. No one knew about those 40 extra pounds that took me so much work to lose. No one knew about my yo-yo dieting over the years. And no one even suspected that I was a junk food junkie of royal proportions.

What did impress me the most about my Kansas neighbors, however, was that these folks came out to the gym like clockwork every day the gym was open to play and get some exercise – no matter that they weren't Twiggy and had to change in the locker room in front of a lot of people. That takes guts, especially since, at their ages, most of them had had some health issues or other, and still had the scars to prove it. From any form of cancer surgeries that left a variety of scars anywhere on the body, to heart attacks and bypass surgery that left some life-long visible roadmaps on their chests. There were pacemakers visible just under the skin, and blood sugar levels being checked by diabetics after each volleyball game. Also, of course there were knee replacements that left angry red stripes down the front of their knees. Of course I brought my own issues: spine and neck scars that reminded me of so many days I had suffered with extreme pain, and so many I still struggled with on a lesser but regular basis.

With this group, they all had something they'd lived through or were still struggling with, including their weight, yet it didn't stop them. And most of them were in their 70's. One was even in her 80's! They must have had some powerful

 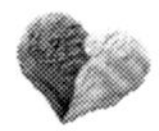

Mojo of their own, is all I can say! They sure didn't use their health issues as excuses.

For me, I really didn't want to add any new owies to my beat-up body, as I needed it to last for as long as possible. I viewed water volleyball as no contact or pounding as we were in waist-deep or higher water. And one could hit the ball (a light-weight beach ball even – not a real volleyball) as many times as you wanted, to get it over the net. Considering that they were mostly retirees, it seemed about as safe as one could get, right?

But despite loving the game and really looking forward to playing as well as hanging out with the players, by January my left shoulder was killing me. It was even screaming at me in the middle of the night, waking me up. Much to my chagrin, I went under the knife again in May to have my shoulder (rotator cuff) fixed. The bad news? I would have to wear a very large, hot, claustrophobic sling for four weeks, and in the heat of the summer, no less. The worst news: I couldn't play volleyball for six months! Certainly didn't see that one coming. I had finally found the perfect situation, and in the blink of an eye it was gone!

So, there I was, unable to do *anything* at the gym for several weeks except for walking on the treadmill or riding the stationary bike, but since the weather was nice enough, I could at least walk outside and walk the dog. However, it's not easy trying to pick up dog poop with one arm in a sling, let me assure you! That took a bit of practice.

And so, I left the treadmill behind and took up daily walks with my dog, who was practically doing cartwheels at this turn of events. When I'd lived in Denver we'd frequented the

80-acre dog park daily, but I'd fallen off that activity in Kansas, where the dog park was about the size of a large postage stamp. That was just too disappointing. And since I'd been busy for weeks with all the unpacking and such, I hadn't really thought about going for walks, as I was exhausted enough.

At least, that is, not until I met some new neighbors who had two big dogs that they walked twice a day. They told me that they walked at least 40 minutes per outing, which could be up to four miles, just to burn off their extra energy. I was impressed. My brain started weighing some ideas. I couldn't do much for several weeks but I could walk. And Larkin would get some exercise too. She could stand to lose a few. Sounded like killing two birds with one stone, to me. So walking became my new volleyball.

We started out at just 30 minutes per day at first, but increasing our time little by little. The hardest part was that I wanted to go at a quick pace to get my heart rate up. She wanted it to be a more typical sniffing, meandering sort of dog walk. I told her she was a slacker and that if she didn't keep up I would have to leave her home. Whether she understood me or not, she got the message and we moved right along. At least most of the time.

It wasn't long before we were up to an hour every day, and it soon became part of our daily routine. Unless the weather made it impossible, you'd see us out there like clockwork. If the weather didn't cooperate, I returned to the treadmill and Larkin just had to miss a day.

And surprise, surprise, my additional pounds slowly began to leave me. I didn't notice at first, as I really didn't see how just walking was going to be enough, but sure enough, I was losing a pound here and there.

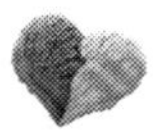

Then, another stroke of luck happened; my daughter came home with a new ice cream she'd discovered called Halo Top – a low-calorie ice cream, but one that didn't taste like it was a diet product, as is usually the case. It also was touted as healthy. What a concept. Apparently social media was spreading the word about it like crazy and it was hard to find it in the grocery stores. Perhaps its followers were hoarding it as it came in? Its spot on the freezer shelves was frequently empty.

Halo Top came in pint containers, like Ben and Jerry's, only with drastically fewer calories. Whereas an entire pint of Ben and Jerry's Cherry Garcia weighed in at 960 calories, Halo Top was a mere 240! I wasn't sure, but I thought I'd died and gone to heaven. Healthy ice cream with the same number of calories as a Snickers candy bar, and would take me longer to polish off than a Snickers bar? What's not to love?

I did a Google search on the frosty treat and found several reviews, with a variety of opinions. But the one that really caught my eye was an article written by a science blogger who, for some reason, decided he was going to eat nothing but Halo Top ice cream for ten days. Yep – five pints of the stuff each day, totaling 1,200 calories per day. A pretty low number in any dieter's book.

I raced through the article that told of his experiences surviving on 50 pints of the stuff for ten days and was I astounded by the results! He lost 10 pounds! Now, mind you, most of us simply couldn't stand eating just ice cream and nothing else for that long. And many folks wouldn't last long on 1,200 calories per day, no matter what the food. But the good news was that in one day's worth of Halo Top and nothing else he consumed 120 grams of protein, only 80 grams of carbs, and 60 grams of fat. Which is pretty good and, if you consider typical junk food, it's certainly better than eating just Snickers bars or Hostess cupcakes for 10 days running!

I was intrigued. Could I do that? I decided I would like to see if I could. I did, however, limit myself to seven days instead of ten. I should certainly have a feel for it by then, I told myself.

I have to admit to eating closer to 75% Halo Top and 25% real food, purely because I did get bored. Not that it wasn't tasty – it was. But somehow my sugar addiction seemed to have calmed down with all the ice cream. First thing I noticed after two or three days; I wasn't even thinking about the chocolate chip cookies I got at the 7-Eleven almost every day, or the carrot cake I loved from the nearby Walmart. Second, amazing as it was, I found that I just wasn't often hungry. A rare situation for me.

Not even the emotional hunger seemed to show its ugly head. That hunger that you know is really conjured up by your mind, not by your stomach actually being empty.

I also noticed I didn't plan ahead for the next binge as I often did. And my usually bloaty stomach had seemed to quiet down and behave normally, which it hadn't done in a while. Interesting, I pondered. Was this all a result of the ice cream?

By the end of my seven days I was down four pounds. That, combined with the daily walking was definitely shaking things up.

I started evolving a new idea or two about dieting. What if, I asked myself, some of this discovery had to do with me not thinking of the ice cream as "cheating" food? I wasn't being bad, eating it. It was just food. What if there was no such

 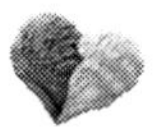

thing as cheating, only eating? And if there was no cheating, there didn't need to be any guilt either – right? Food was just food and I made choices every day about which foods and how much I put in my mouth.

I thought about this concept. Guilt had always been the real devil for me and for so many other friends I knew who were struggling with weight. I had a ying-yang thing going on. Every time I put a morsel of forbidden food in my mouth, that little devil would appear on my shoulder, urging me to eat whatever and however much of the forbidden tidbits were calling me. And the little angel – my cheerleader, my Miss Mojo on my other shoulder – was kindly reminding me of how much better I was going to feel later if I put the food down and walked away instead.

I got to thinking, sure, there would be times when I would overeat – and not just bad foods either. But what if I could change my attitude about food? What if I looked at all those horrible things that I still ate every day as just *food,* not *forbidden food*? Could I change my perspective about food itself? What if, when I ate that particular negative food, despite my little cheerleader's urging me not to, I *didn't* feel horrible or guilty about it like I normally did? What if I felt all right about it? Just how different would that make dieting for me?

What if the key was that I could eat *anything* I wanted but just not in the amount I was used to? In other words, I could eat any food at all – even the ones I had labeled "bad." But I just couldn't eat a ton of it? And, I could eat cookies, but if I wanted to eat more than just cookies that day, then I had to limit myself to two cookies and had to count them in my calories. I could eat a shake from Sonic, which would be counted as my entire dinner, and therefore I wouldn't also eat an appetizer at the same sitting. I could eat my favorite fudge from the local grocery store every day, if I wanted, but I had to do so while counting calories and fitting it within my allotted calories for the day. And if I wanted a glass of wine, I'd likely have to skip the chocolates that I'd been thinking of having for dessert. Or another option would be that I could have half a serving of each, which could still fit within my parameters.

The pieces of my project started coming together I started making some notes ...

One was that I had this interesting thought about the concept of cheating itself. It occurred to me that usually when someone cheats, they do something bad to achieve something they perceive is good (something they want). For example, if they cheat on a test, they do so to get a better grade. If they cheat on their taxes, they do something bad (lie to Uncle Sam) in the hopes of getting more money back on their taxes. And, if they cheat on a diet, they do something bad (eat those bad foods) – but what is the *good part* they get back? Honestly, I didn't see that there was one, other than a few minutes of pleasure. Instead, there was guilt! That didn't seem like a good thing to me. Where was the benefit? So I decided that the whole concept of cheating had to go.

Instead, it had to be about making choices and taking responsibility for them.

I continued brainstorming ... if I decided to overeat and exceed the number of calories I allotted myself in a day, then it was simply my choice and I was telling myself one of two things: 1.) That I made a choice that was not in sync with my

 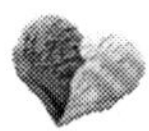

goals and I would simply pick myself up and dust myself off and put that choice behind me, and go forth or 2.) that my intention regarding weight loss (at least at that moment) was not at 100 percent. I was simply not ready to commit to take on the job at that time. And that was OK too. It was just up to me to be honest with myself. And quit wasting my time and energy dieting if my subconscious really hadn't bought into it.

Moreover, I remembered a concept I'd learned a long time ago, about the expression, "I can't." Whenever, for example, I use the words, "I can't" lose weight, I've already convinced myself from the get-go that it is simply not possible. And it's not in my control. It's like I'm a marionette and someone else is pulling my strings and running my life. And I have no say in my decisions or outcomes.

However, if I substitute the expression, "I choose," or "I choose not," instead of "I can't," I take my power back and my life back. I either choose to lose the weight or I choose not to lose the weight. I choose to overeat, or I choose not to overeat. I choose to exercise or I don't. But saying "I can't ____________" (fill in the blank with whatever your action is, for example, "I can't exercise, I can't eat healthy, I can't live without chocolate") is simply not an option. For with those words you've sealed your fate before even getting started.

And when it comes to excuses – which goes right along with "I can't," I had to throw all of them out as well. For even despite all the physical issues I'd been battling for years, I could still at least walk, couldn't I? And I was noticing in just a short amount of time that walking was working, albeit slowly but surely. So, no excuses. Period. Sure, modifications were possible, like the many things I had to do somewhat differently at Rancho Cortez. (Wall pushups versus kneeling pushups.) But I still worked out with all my other gym rats for the same number of hours they did. And even pushed the edge of my envelope on Enchanted Rock, when my gut reaction was to automatically pull out one of my excuses. So, no. No excuses allowed.

Then, I remembered there was the power statement: Tryin's Lyin'. "There is no try, only do or don't do," Yoda reminded me. If I couldn't visualize it happening, if I didn't believe in myself, if I was only willing to "try," then I was doomed to fail. Instead, I needed to set a clear goal with powerful visual words. I wrote in my journal: I WILL weigh 148 pounds, my high school weight, within two months. I envisioned myself in the bikini I wore after all my months of working out and losing weight for the wedding.

Along with this, I had a new acronym: W.A.L.K., which stood for "What All Losers Know." (Of course that meant weight losers, not the other kind of losers where you put a big L with your thumb and first finger on your forehead!). Nearly everyone can walk. It takes no special equipment, gym membership, talent, knowledge, skill, or strength. And even if the weather was bad and you couldn't afford a gym membership you could walk in most malls and still get a workout. Even folks who use medical walkers full time can oftentimes walk more than they routinely do. I was a walker-user several times after my various back and knee surgeries, so I know it takes a bit more work, for sure, to have to drag the damned thing all over the place. But if a little bit of work could lead you to getting healthier, getting stronger, and

 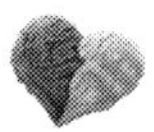

maybe even dropping a few pounds, might it not be worth it? (Obviously check with your doctor first before starting any new weight loss plan.)

***

I wrote all those concepts in my new journal with those powerful words and expressions that were to become my tools to staying on track. I re-read them every day. I still use some form of most of them even now. They are timeless tools every dieter would be wise to make part of his or her daily mantra or meditation.

And then, having put my mental side of this battle in order, it was time to face the details (where that devil resides).

I still had to remember the basic lessons I learned in preparation for the wedding ... weight loss is pure math. (Once you get past the psychology factors: guilt and all that.) It boils down to calories-in versus calories-out. Whatever I ate in excess would go to storage. Yep – I loved it on my lips, but hated it on my hips! Whenever I ate less than what I burned, I lost weight. Whenever I ate more than I burned, it stuck like glue. The last key factor was deciding how many calories I was willing to allow myself each day.

Looking back to my pre-wedding successful tracking, I was hovering most of the time around 1,800-2,000 calories as my maximum intake and burning around 2,500-2,800, which wasn't bad. However, after reading about the guy who lived on five Halo Tops per day, which was only 1,200 calories, I decided I could probably cut down on my intake, especially since, unlike my pre-wedding phase where I was working out like a fiend, I was now limited to only walking. I decided to aim for about 1,400 calories per day as my goal in the losing phase. I could add more to that once I hit the 148, but would have to experiment with just how much more I could eat without gaining any back. That's where a tracker can be a big help.

I was ready. Larkin was ready. My Misfit was ready. And there was plenty of Halo Top in the freezer – not to be lived on full time, but to provide me with my fix to my still-quite-alive sugar addiction. Mind you, I wasn't suggesting that I couldn't lose weight without the Halo Top. That was just one item in my personal arsenal. Normally, I couldn't keep anything sugary in bulk in my house, but somehow, in my mind, I'd already labeled the diet ice cream as "food," not "bad stuff," and I guess because I'd had my fill of it for those seven days, I didn't crave it any longer. Although I did usually have one pint or so per day.

I also reaffirmed that there's no such thing as cheatin' and I could eat whatever the heck I wanted … but by the end of the day I had to stay at or under 1,400 calories.

My personal goal was a lofty one. My 100 percent intention was to get back to my high school track team weight of 148 pounds by the time I finished writing this book! It was going to be a reach but after what I had seen was possible as far back as the weeks prior to Shaun's wedding, as well as just the small results that were starting to add up just walking, I believed, for the first time in years, that I could do it.

And if I could do it, Larkin could do it too. I had adopted her from a shelter several years ago. She'd been found wandering the streets of Denver, with a new haircut and a collar with

 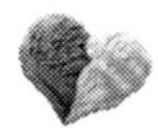

her name on it, but no contact info. So obviously someone had taken care of her fairly recently, but no one seemed to be looking for her now. She was starving and weighed in at 13 pounds at about a year old. I'd had several dogs over the years, and most of the time only one at a time, so I would always keep their food dish full, letting them eat as they wanted. Well, that idea wasn't going to work with this little girl as she'd instantly inhale the entire bowl every time I filled it. I guess she was afraid the food might disappear again, so she'd best fill up while it was around. So, it became apparent that I'd need to put her on a specific amount of food once her weight stabilized, or she'd be at risk of becoming overweight herself. At that point she was about 17 pounds, a perfect weight for her.

However, I did feed her occasional dog treats, being careful not to give her too many and instead gave her rawhide bones; the doggie version of low-cal snacks.

About that time, I had gone to Rancho Cortez for two weeks and I sent Larkin to my favorite dog sitter family, who loved her to death. They lived on a small ranch with horses and dogs and cats and goats and all sorts of fun things to do. And they also had really yummy dog treats! And Larkin, with that poor little face that said, "I was starving once and I'll never forget that awful feeling. So can I please have another dog treat since my mom is gone? I miss her terribly." And she'd look at them with those pleading, brown, sad eyes and no one could possibly resist.

I came home from Rancho Cortez down four pounds. She came home from the dog sitter's weighing twenty! It looked like we both had our work cut out for us!

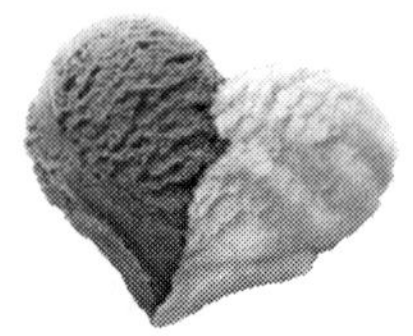

CHAPTER 28

Butt! Butt! Butt!

So Larkin and I picked up the pace, and for a few weeks I even cut her dog food back just a wee bit as well. She's a tiny dog, so gets about 3/4 of a cup of kibble per day. I've had many people suggest I'm starving the poor girl, but if you hadn't noticed, a huge number of dogs are morbidly obese in this culture as well! She didn't need to be one of them.

I'd given myself two months to write the book because my goal was to have books available for readers by the first of the year when New Year's resolutions for weight loss are at their peak. It takes several months for a book to go from a manuscript to a real book you can hold in your hands. In fact, starting the writing project the first of July was still unlikely that I could meet that goal even if I did finish the book in two months, but what the heck? I'm the eternal optimist. Plus, I absolutely love the writing process. And I have always performed best when under a deadline!

I set the goal of reaching 148 pounds at the same time as finishing the writing as just an extra challenge! No small feat accomplishing either one, much less both. And so I immersed myself in both of them, crawling out of bed at 6:30 a.m. when

 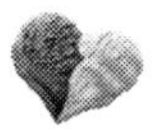

I so didn't want to. But with the temperatures often in the 90's with ungodly humidity, we had to get out and walk as soon as the sun came up. Ugh. By the time we walked in the door every day I was drenched in sweat and headed immediately to the shower.

Then for the rest of the day and evening I lived in front of my computer, hoping the stories and the facts might all tie together by the end.

The days raced by. As I wrote my daily numbers in my journal and on the calendar each day, I saw things starting to take place. The number of pages in the manuscript started climbing nicely as my daily meeting with the scales showed the slightest of improvements. Larkin didn't get a journal because first of all, her food didn't change day to day. She got her measured dog food and I was very stingy with the dog cookies. Plus, her scales were at the vet's but I did have to take her for shots and such a couple of times and I smiled each time she weighed in as her numbers were moving in the right direction as well, although only by tenths of a pound. I could almost see a waist appearing on her physique if I used my imagination a wee bit.

As for goal number one, MISSION ACCOMPLISHED! The book was done. I wrapped up the last chapter at the end of 6 weeks, with room to spare!

As for the 148 pounds, I hit 149.5 this week and if all goes well, I'm pretty sure I'll reach it as well. Just how long I'll stay that low, I really don't know. On the one hand, I'd be pleased as punch to keep that number as my baseline. Yet Miss Mojo has been suggesting that 146 would mean that I'd be down an even 50 pounds since my heaviest time. And 50 has a nice ring to it. I guess you'll have to stay tuned to my Facebook page to see where else this journey takes me. And by the way, my legs are getting some awesome muscles too!

And Little Larkin – she's down a whopping 3 pounds! That doesn't sound like much, but that's 15 percent! And 15 percent on a human male who weighs 200 pounds is 30 pounds! So she won, hands down, for the biggest percentage of weight loss! And she also won a few more daily cookies to keep her in maintenance mode. She wasn't complaining. After all, she gets an hour walk every day and increased food in her bowl! I wish I was her.

***

We all have a thousand excuses why we believe we can't lose weight. No time. Can't afford a gym membership. Don't have anyone to work out with. Embarrassed to get naked in the locker room.

Well, let me remind you that if anyone has legitimate excuses it was me. Count them: Three back surgeries. One neck surgery. Both knees replaced. One shoulder surgery. And Parkinson's disease. Just looking at all those legitimate excuses on paper should have given me a doctor's excuse to opt out of any of the physical things I was still doing. But despite it all, I could still walk. In fact, our little hour walk every day averages nearly 24 miles per week – almost a marathon! It doesn't sound so little now, does it?

Looking back, it has been quite a journey. From my high school track team days through 40 years of yo-yo dieting and weight gain and loss, through the experiences at a fat farm

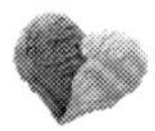

and becoming a gym rat, to dropping forty pounds for the wedding and more. Here are some of the lessons I gleaned on my travels ...

I don't have to starve myself to lose weight. But I do have to understand calories-in versus calories-out and what portions really look like. If I can count and spend a few minutes per day tracking my food, it's easier to stay the course.

I can eat *anything* I want, just not *everything* I want. If I want to eat pizza all day I can, I just need to make sure I don't exceed my calorie max for the day. If I'm craving 600 calories of ice cream for breakfast? No worries, I just have to figure out how I'm going to fit that into my remaining 800 calories for the rest of the day.

My revised view of cheating and eating and good food and bad food is something that helps me whether I'm actively taking steps to lose weight or simply maintain it. I don't feel as though I have to hide my junk food eating from anyone anymore. If I am going to Thanksgiving dinner where I know the average number of calories consumed on such a meal is well over 3,000, I'll just plan ahead and eat light on both the day before as well as the day after the holiday, so that I can still eat what I want on Turkey Day and not wake up feeling guilty about it the next day.

Plus, no matter what, I PROMISE not to let Great Aunt Matilda talk me into taking home ANY leftovers, no matter how yummy they are! For the same reason I never bring home bags of cookies. Or boxes of granola bars. Or any of my other favorite yummies that come in bulk. I just KNOW if they're on my shelves, they're just too easy. And too readily available. (Remember the Klondike Bars?) I just don't need the temptation.

My improved knowledge and understanding of calories and portions keep me aware of what I'm eating and what choices are smartest for me. I understand that a Dairy Queen Blizzard is not an appetizer to a meal, it IS the meal! Bernie taught me well that 80 percent of weight loss is the food and only 20 percent is the exercise. In other words – I CAN'T OUTRUN THE FORK!

My brain is always doing calorie calculations, whether I'm going to the movies tonight and am planning on eating an entire bucket of popcorn all by myself, or if it's order-in pizza night with friends. I am totally aware of what I put in my mouth. That's my trick to holding my weight steady. And I'll tell you something – it's a whole lot easier doing that than being in active diet mode!

Whenever possible, I plan my largest meal of the day first, then fill in the rest. For example, if I know I'm having pizza tonight, that helps me make lighter choices throughout the day, knowing that my pizza dinner can easily use up a thousand calories or more. Otherwise, if I'm just not paying attention it's so easy to find myself at dinner time with no calories left and a rumbling in my empty tummy all night.

 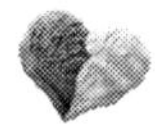

My sugar/junk food addiction has not gone away, but I have learned to balance it with eating something healthy every day. I also take vitamins to help my body get what it needs that I'm not giving it by eating the non-nutritious meals I frequently eat.

I must never forget that, if I want to keep the weight off, I have to keep after it every day. It must be a lifestyle, not a diet that ends after a certain number of weeks. In fact, for some people, losing the weight is the easy part. Keeping it off is much harder. But like anything else, it gets easier as you do it each day.

I don't have to be a gym rat or a jock to lose weight. I don't even have to work out hard. But I do have to move every day for at least an hour. Walk, swim, bike, play tennis, whatever. While I lost weight at the gym (after several months of not losing) and a few at the fitness bootcamp, I didn't need to spend lots of money on my quest. In the long run, my easiest, most consistent, cheapest weight loss occurred when all I was allowed to do was walk.

Having a partner to share my weight loss journey with makes the road so much easier. Whether I partner up with a friend or family member, or even one of the online chat groups, I don't have to go through this alone. Plus, having someone to celebrate with when I reach each new goal doubles the fun!

Yet, the best part in my crazy love/hate relationship with food has obviously been finally finding something that worked for me. And realizing that weight loss, just like weight gain, doesn't happen overnight.

***

This has been my story. Some ups. Some downs. Lots of excuses. Lots of denial. Many lessons learned. And many yet to come.

You have your own story as well. Mine isn't anything unusual. Whether you have fought your weight all your life or like me, or it caught up with you sooner or later, your story affects the way you feel about food.

You can let your story make you stronger with your own little Miss Mojo (or other inner messenger) or you can use it as an excuse why you simply can't lose weight. Why you believe diets don't work. Why you think you can never be as thin as the skinny girl who looks like she's always been skinny and can eat whatever she wants and still doesn't gain a pound.

Because we're all different, what works for each of us will vary as well. You don't have to do what I did. Find something that's right for you. The important thing is that you choose something you can live with and something you can believe in. And it needs to be something you can implement for a lifetime.

Unless your intention to lose weight is 100 percent, then don't even start a weight-loss program or you will only make yourself miserable. And losing weight because someone else wants you to is the other sure fire way to ensure yourself a bad outcome. Remember – 'Tryin's Lyin'. Don't ever try to lose

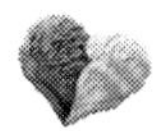

weight. Either make the commitment, or just put it off for another time when you are ready.

In addition, addictions of any kind – drugs, alcohol, sugar, you name it – can be tied to deeper issues than just seeking that satisfying rush. Sometimes professional help is necessary to help us break through some issues that are keeping us stuck. So keep your mind open to various types of therapy and support that could help you and your own Miss Mojo find a healthier, happier life.

You deserve it.

Epilogue

I was wrapping up this book when I happened to run into someone I hadn't seen in a long time. We got to talking and her story left me humbled ... and motivated. My wish is that it may do the same for you ...

It happened at a cowboy dance bar in Denver where I was meeting up with a guy buddy one night. He was a regular there, so had his groupies who filled up his dance card pretty quickly, giving me time to look over all the folks in their cowboy/cowgirl outfits: boots, hats, belt buckles, you get the picture. *People-watching*, my mom used to call it. This bar wasn't a place where I hung out a lot, so I really didn't expect to run into anyone I knew. Suddenly, a vivacious woman, likely late 40's or a little better, slid onto the bar stool next to me.

"Mary Jo!" she exclaimed, a bit out of breath as she'd apparently seen me and dashed across the dance floor, hoping not to get run over by the masses.

She was fashionably thin and dressed in her cute cowgirl dance outfit. She had soft, wavy brown curls, that bounced when she walked. Vibrant brown eyes. And a sense of excitement and anticipation – as though life was a game and she was a winning player. I didn't recognize her but her voice was really familiar. So I kept watching her as she spoke and prayed that her very distinctive voice was going to make the connection soon so I wouldn't have to look like an idiot for long.

"How ARE you?" she began. "Gosh, I haven't seen you in years! You look great!"

Nope. Still didn't know who she was. I kept encouraging her to take the lead in the conversation by asking her some broad questions that still let her talk. "So how are you? And the family?" I asked, somewhat tentatively.

She filled me in about the kids. (All grown up.) How she was still at the same job. How she and her boyfriend came here nearly every week and why she was so surprised to see me here, since she hadn't before.

At long last, I had to fess up and I told her that I still couldn't place her.

"Oh, gosh. I forgot. You haven't seen me since ... " She looked embarrassed, yet at the same time, happy.

"Since what?" I asked. Definitely curious.

"Since my weight loss. I lost 120 pounds last year and now so many people don't recognize me." She waited to see if I could figure it out then, but nope, I still had no clue.

"It's me, MJ. It's Jane from the days of the kids in Pony Club."

My brain tried to apply it's best facial recognition app and while that name and the voice were making the connection, my brain still couldn't believe it was the same woman. She was tall like me, vivacious, high energy, happy, and looked 10 years younger than I'd remembered. Holy moly!

We chatted for some time about her weight loss and how she'd gone the traditional route – eating healthy, getting rid of all processed foods, cooking from scratch, portion control, low fat, low carb, no sugar or salt, and whole grains. And how, after making these changes, her body could no longer tolerate high calorie, high fat foods, except for the occasional dark chocolate! She did confess to still being hooked on diet soda, however.

Of course, her life had changed with her weight loss as well. She was certainly happier with herself and less self-conscious about her body, she added. She also just felt healthier. She told me how her youngest daughter was about to get married and how her special needs son, a young man with Down's Syndrome in his late 20's, even had a girlfriend. She introduced me to her long-term boyfriend and I watched them spend much of the night dancing the night away, smiling, definitely smitten with each other, and definitely enjoying life.

Wow! I said to myself. Now that's a woman with no if's, ands, or butts! (Pun intended!) She'd obviously, for whatever reason, decided that she wanted to be one of those thin people. She'd set her intention, taken the necessary steps, and stuck to her plan as more than just a diet. It was a lifestyle for her.

Now, I thought to myself, she's going to be one of those skinny people that overweight people hate, because they think she was born skinny and never had to worry about eating whatever she wanted, never knowing just how much work she did to get to where she was today, and every day that came after. Boy, I knew that feeling.

I decided to ask her one last question when she took a break from the dance floor. "So, Jane, what made you decide to lose the weight? That's usually the hardest step for anyone. And if it's someone else who's pushing you to lose weight and you're not doing it for yourself, it always ends in disaster."

"You're absolutely right," she confirmed. "Well, I got a major wake up call. I'd gone in for a routine physical and when the doctor looked at my blood work he informed me that I was pre-diabetic and said if I didn't change my eating habits and lose some of the weight fast, that full-fledged diabetes was waiting for me."

"How frightening," I empathized. My mom had lived with diabetes and I knew it well.

She continued, "I spend a lot of time working with the special needs and disabled community," she explained. "And it struck me that this was a disease I could choose to have, or not choose to have, unlike a lot of the kids and parents I worked with who did not have a choice in their disabilities. I felt fortunate enough to get to make that choice myself. But even more important than all that, I realized that I had to stay as healthy as I could so that I would be around to take care of my son Jake for as long as possible."

I think my heart skipped a beat there. To her it was simply reality. To those of us not in a position like that, it was an incredibly unselfish act of a loving mother.

"That was my royal kick in the butt." She tried to smile, but I knew it must have been hard to talk about. "The worst part about it was that I never saw myself as that heavy and neither did my kids. I show them photos of me from back then now and they don't believe it's me!"

"I know," I nodded. "I posted a picture of me when I weighed 40 pounds more a few years back and people ask me, "Did we know you then?" (They did.) "They surely didn't remember me like that."

"The last part of my motivation to lose it was that I had been divorced for several years after some pretty difficult ones. And finally, I had gotten rid of so many old emotions that kept the weight on. I had done my healing and growing. I felt free."

Then she flashed me a huge, truly happy smile and said, "I became the person I was supposed to be."

***

Who are you supposed to be?

What excuses have you been hiding behind?

How different would your life be if you were thin?

The choice is yours.

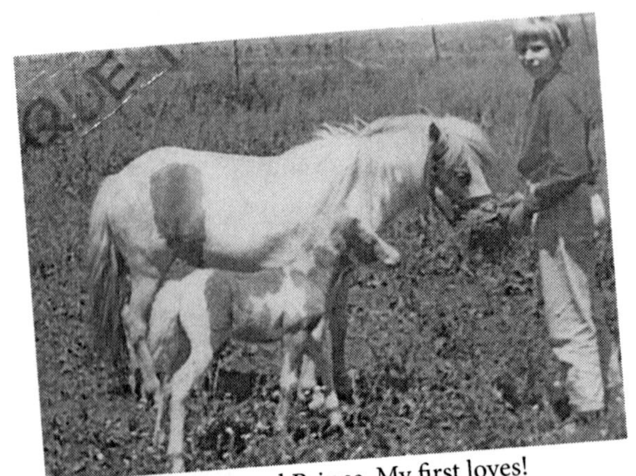

Queenie and Prince. My first loves!

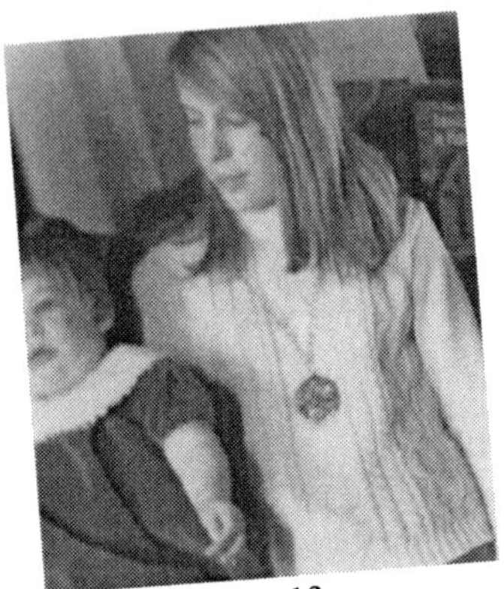

Age 13

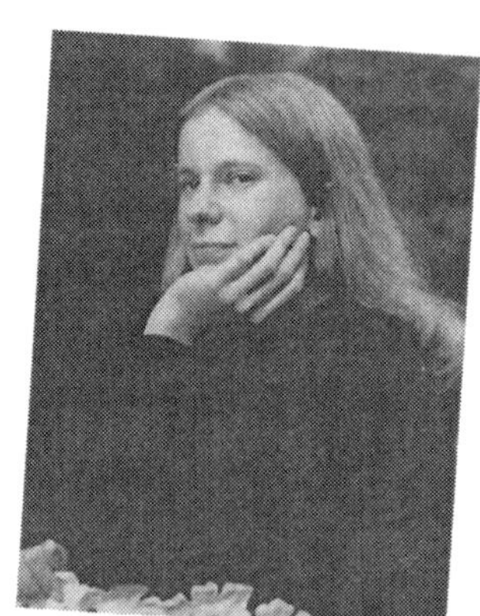

Senior class photo

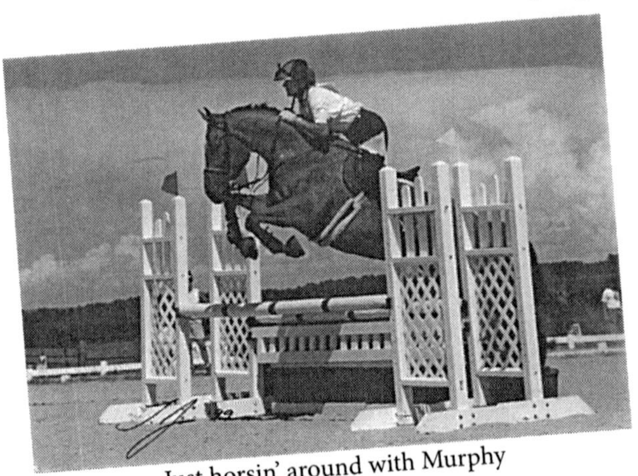

Just horsin' around with Murphy

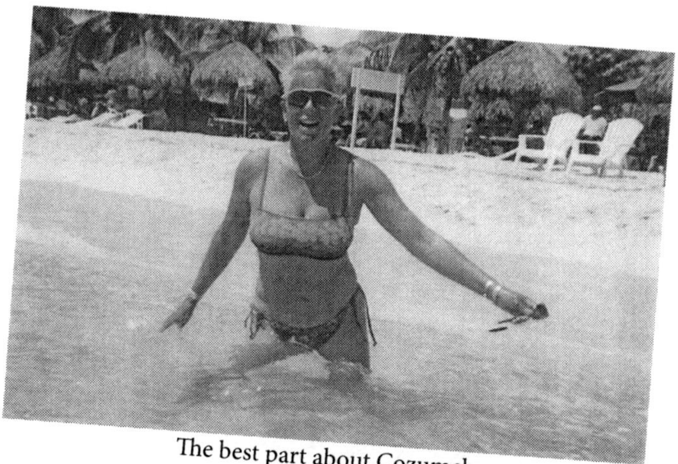
The best part about Cozumel

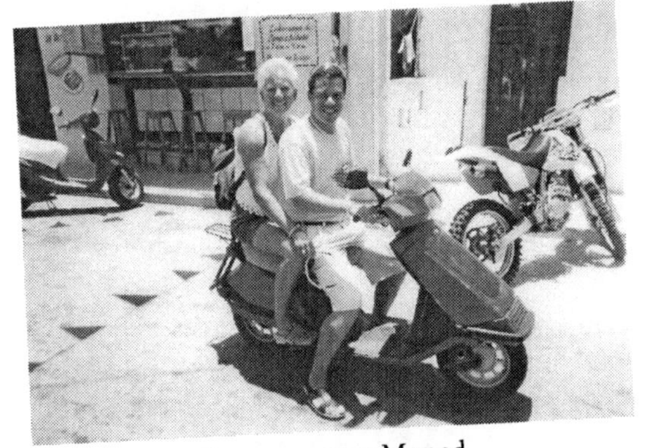
Romance on a Moped

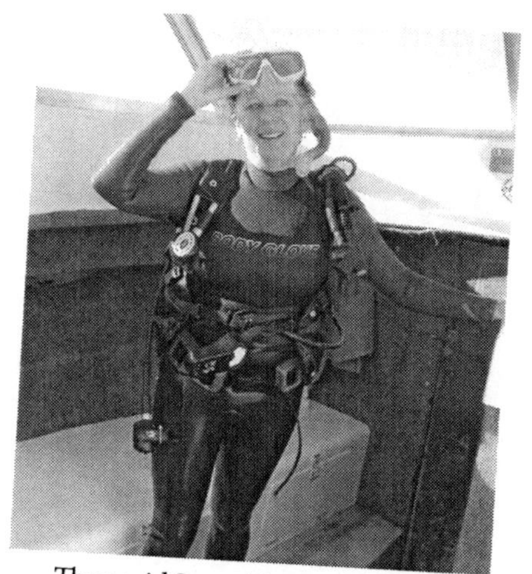
They said I was like a mermaid!

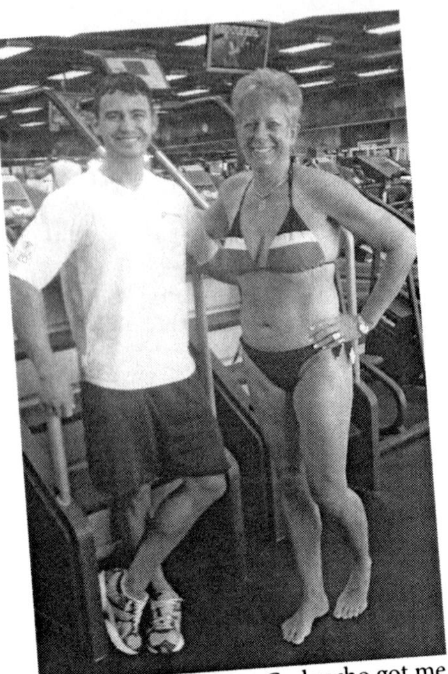
Thanks to my trainer, Cody who got me in shape in the nick of time!

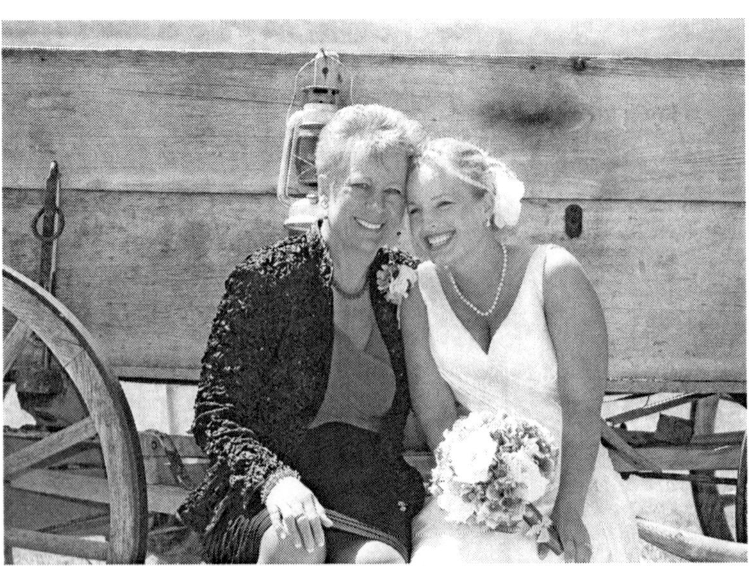
Proud Mama of the bride with my amazing daughter, Shaun

Acknowledgments

It truly does take a team to birth a book. No author can do it alone. As such, I'd like to thank all my amazing team members who helped me on this journey ...

First, to all my friends who encouraged me in so many ways. From Rene Ryman who nursed me back to health after shoulder surgery slowed me down in my writing goals! She also always pushes me to write, as she says I'm "on fire" when I have a new writing project in full swing!

To my water volleyball buddies who welcomed me to Topeka last year – you'll never know just how much your friendship and kindness helped me as I transitioned to a new home. And how you quite accidentally sent me on the path of writing this book.

To several folks who actually read the entire manuscript, front to back, in a super timely manner, offering comments, editorial advice, and insights. Thanks to Mary Andreni, Nancy Stern, Bunny Cornfeld, Marjorie Collins, Becky Drager, Carol Pluta and Mary Carwile.

To John Kremer for his great ideas – not only about the cover but for his marketing ideas as well.

To Judith Briles, The Book Shepard, for teaching me how to produce a great book!

Then there are all the technical folks: My incredible graphic artist, Nick Zelinger, who turned my piecemeal thoughts into an amazing cover and laid out the book beautifully.

To Barb Munson, my amazing editor, who let my voice shine through despite my unconventional writing style.

To Margie Le Bow for that great back cover photo. You beautifully captured my dog and me in that picture.

To Teri Koren for sharing your story with me. What a powerful message we can all use!

To my amazing daughter Shaun, who said, "There are enough self-help, diet books out there, Mom. Write YOUR story." What great advice that was! I so appreciate your unconditional love and support.

Of course I have to thank my canine gal-pal, Larkin, not only for her role in various parts of the story but as well for being my 24-hour companion – especially during all those nights that I kept writing until the wee hours, when she'd have likely preferred that we went to bed much earlier. Who also had to learn to walk fast rather than meander to inhale the smells on our walks. I know that was a sacrifice!

And as always, to God above, for all the words and images you provided when I began with none. You truly do work in mysterious and wonderful ways!

About The Author

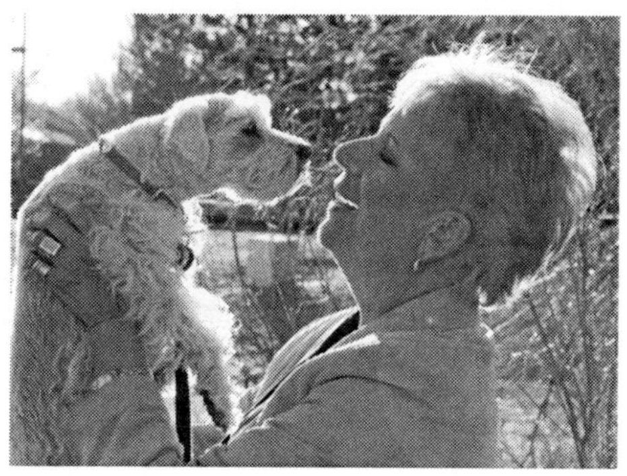

Mary Jo Fay is a speaker, coach, columnist, screen writer, and award-winning author of 6 books, both fiction and non-fiction. Educated as a nurse, she never dreamed that her career would lead her to nursing people's relationships – including the ones they have with themselves. Her previous books include non-fiction self-help works: *Get Out of Your Boxx, When Your Perfect Partner Goes Perfectly Wrong, The Seven Secrets of Love, and Please Dear, Not Tonight – The Truth About Women and Sex*. She has also penned an erotic thriller, *Blatant Deception*. In this, her latest book, *No Cheatin', Just Eatin'*, she focuses on our oftentimes crazy love/hate relationships with food.

Admitting to being a Junk Food Junkie herself, she invites you to join her on her journey of 40 years of yo-yo dieting and binge eating to discovering how she really could eat anything and still lose weight. She's glad to share her success with you, hoping that you may find yourself in part, if not all, of this book.

She lives in Kansas near family and friends, and of course – with her dog, Larkin.

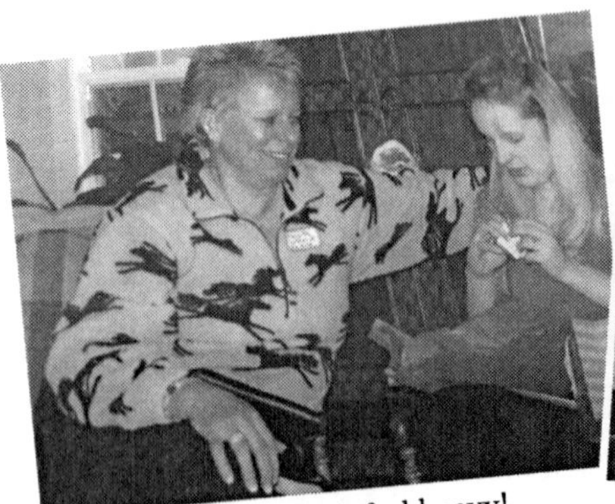

Funny - I didn't feel heavy!

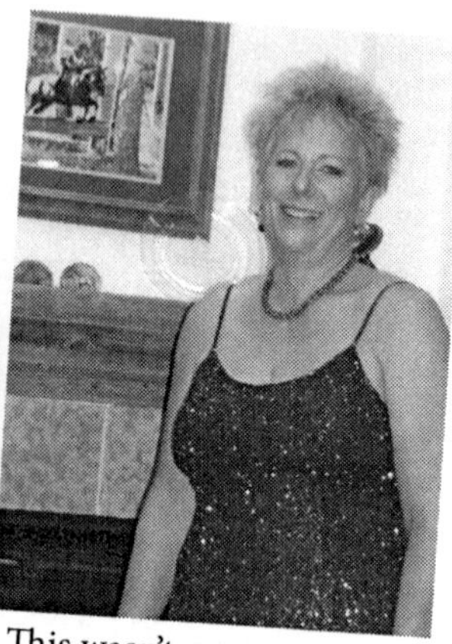

This wasn't even my max.
Not long after I couldn't
fit in this dress either!

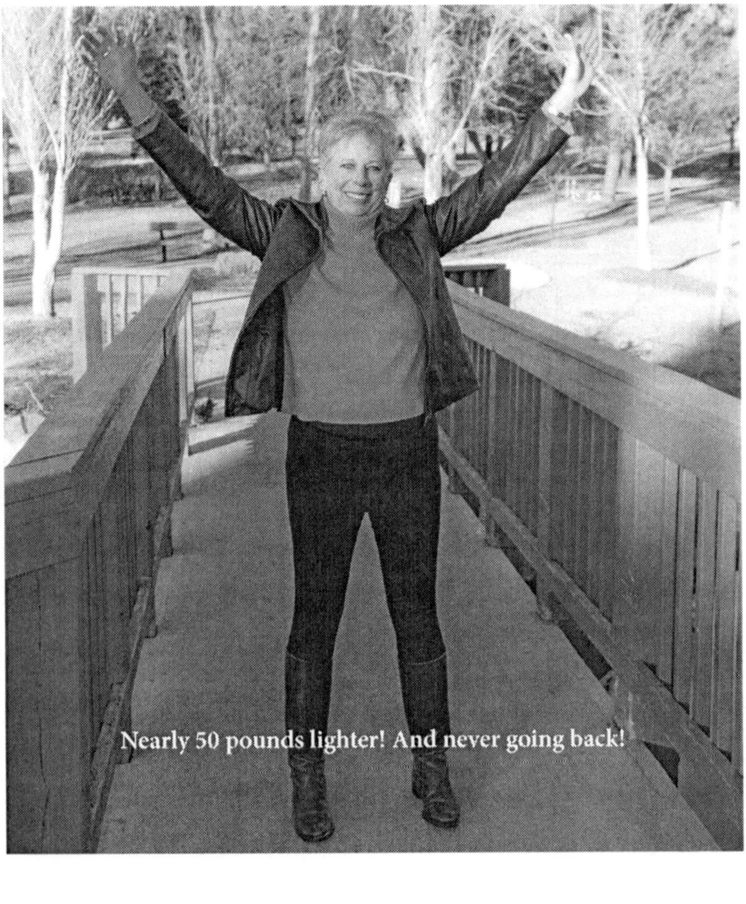

Nearly 50 pounds lighter! And never going back!

CPSIA information can be obtained
at www.ICGtesting.com
Printed in the USA
FFOW03n0202300117
31771FF

9 780998 176406